Advanced Praise for *Perfect M*

*"While there are many books on maternal depression, **Perfect Mothers Get Depressed** distinguishes itself by exposing the association between women who relentlessly strive for perfection and depression, particularly during the vulnerable postpartum period. Dr. Kimberly Thompson does a beautiful job elucidating very complex concepts by presenting examples and analogies that make the information clear and easy to understand. Her keys to change offer precise and evidence-based guidance. Women and their families will find great comfort and essential insight if they read this book while navigating the challenges of postpartum depression."*

Karen Kleiman, MSW, LCSW
Director, The Postpartum Stress Center
Author, *Therapy and the Postpartum Woman*

*"Kimberly Thompson brings a fresh and thoughtful perspective to our understanding of postpartum illness. She skillfully captures the essence of new mothers' experiences of depression, recognizing that the story of a woman's life is embedded in her symptoms and that understanding her whole story leads to healing. **Perfect Mothers Get Depressed** is a welcome addition to the catalogue of books on perinatal mood disorders."*

Diana Lynn Barnes, PsyD
Editor, *Women's Reproductive Mental Health Across the Lifespan* (Springer, 2014)

"This book by Dr. Thompson is remarkable for including state of the science findings regarding depression's causes and treatments. Simultaneously, the author presents the material in a lively and engaging authentic voice that carries authority without pretentiousness. I will recommend this book to every pregnant woman I know. The information is salient, important and accessible. Bravo to Dr. Thompson on this fine work."

Debra Bendell Estroff, PhD

KIMBERLY D. THOMPSON, PhD

Perfect Mothers Get Depressed

Why Trying to Be Perfect and Please Everyone
Increases Your Risk of Postpartum Depression

Praeclarus Press, LLC

www.PraeclarusPress.com

Praeclarus Press, LLC
2504 Sweetgum Lane
Amarillo, Texas 79124 USA
806-367-9950
www.PraeclarusPress.com

DISCLAIMER
The information contained in this publication is advisory only and is not intended to replace sound clinical judgment or individualized patient care. The author disclaims all warranties, whether expressed or implied, including any warranty as the quality, accuracy, safety, or suitability of this information for any particular purpose.

ISBN: 978-1-939807-30-4

Cover Design: Ken Tackett
Acquisition & Development: Kathleen Kendall-Tackett
Copy Editing: Chris Tackett
Layout & Design: Nelly Murariu
Operations: Scott Sherwood

TABLE OF CONTENTS

CHAPTER 4

**Acting Depressed: Relationship Behaviors and
the Perpetuation of Depression**

CHAPTER 5

**The Keys to Change: Challenging Your Depression,
Changing Your Patterns**

CHAPTER 6

Creating an Anchor Within: Practices to Combat Depression

Dedication

To Doug, who has always believed that I could do anything I wanted to do, and to all my babies, who are now all grown up.

Foreword by
Charles D. Thompson, MD, FACOG

Many books, papers, treatises, research papers, and other documents are written and published on various subjects, including postpartum depression. However, very few are called "game changers," "enlightening," or "paradigm shifting." The content of this book comes from not only research from real-live patients who had postpartum depression, but also from a lifetime of experience as a daughter, wife, mother, and friend to many other mothers with the same affliction. Dr. Thompson's work has so impressed the psychological community, that graduate schools and post-graduate fellows have asked her to impart her knowledge and wisdom of this subject to their psychology students. Dr. Thompson had her doctoral thesis published in a well-respected international psychological journal, and subscribers read her work so often that it became the third most downloaded article of 2014 for the journal. I am truly amazed that all this important work and recognition came from the woman that I fell in love with and married 30 years ago, that I still know as Kim.

Kim did not always have an affinity for psychology, however. She grew up as the only daughter of a Houston school teacher and stay-at-home mother, who had a deep affinity for music. She graduated 7th in her high school class, and went on to Southwestern University in Georgetown, TX, and ultimately received her Bachelor of Music in Christian Education. I grabbed on to her rising star before it even twinkled, and we were married in 1985. She then worked at a church while I was going through medical school. We ultimately had three children and adopted another from Romania. Although

I was trained and practicing medicine in obstetrics and gynecology, I did not recognize the symptoms of postpartum depression in my own wife. She struggled, and ultimately overcame the dark shadow of guilt and shame that often comes with parenting small children, without help from her spouse or parents, all of whom loved her, but did not understand the issues behind her dysfunction.

Although we did not understand her depression, Kim knew that she was feeling inadequate for a reason, and she determined to study this problem. After 14 years of being a superb, but troubled mother, she embarked on her second academic career. It took her another 12 years of study and work, but Kim received her doctorate in Psychology in 2012.

Many times, we are not able to see the forest due to all the trees in the way. We have all heard this euphemism, but you don't understand it until you are really there. Depression has been described has being in a deep, dark place and not knowing where to turn or how to get out, very much like being in the *Schwarzwald* in Germany, or the Piney Woods in East Texas. In order to get out, a woman must learn to survive in the environment in which she finds herself, and cope with the everyday stressors that lie before her. Eventually, she finds a path that leads to light and fresh air, and even though she may have to bring some of the baggage with her, she is finally able to engage in her community again and feel the love of other people. The fact is that most people are able to find their way out, eventually. However, a guide can help you get to your destination faster, with less trauma, and the best guides are the ones who have been there themselves. Dr. Thompson shows you how to navigate through the forest of despair and shame to come out on the other side, with life and hope for the future.

Kim (Dr. Thompson, to y'all) has taught me most of what I know about depression, which is far more than what the medical books ever taught me, and I know that she can teach other physicians and nurses the essentials of diagnosing and treating depression. However, we have to realize that some cures don't come in a pill, but some require changing the thought processes, attitudes, and coping skills of those that are afflicted. I have been amazed at the difference that psychological counseling has had in my patients, which lasts for the long term.

As a husband and father, I recommend reading this book to try to understand what your wife, girlfriend, mother, daughter, sister, or aunt is going through in order to be a positive influence as part of the solution to the problem of depression. It will enlighten and encourage you to see that your loved one can get better and happier.

Lastly, I want to say how proud I am of my dear wife for this work. We never dreamed it would be so important. When we were married, Kim told me that she wanted to do great things for God. Well folks, here it is!

Acknowledgments

I would like to acknowledge the contributions of each of the following people to this work:

Dr. Debra Bendell-Estroff, who has been a remarkable mentor and guide, in conducting the research this book is based upon and beyond.

Dr. Kathleen Kendall-Tackett, who also gave invaluable advice and guidance in conducting and presenting this research.

Dr. Ray Hawkins, who insured that every detail of the research was attended to properly.

Dr. Charles Thompson, Dr. Malissia Zapata, Dr. Marie Hollis, Dr. Teresa Kowalczyk, Kim Katchinska, and *Frankie Haddock,* the obstetrician-gynecologists and certified nurse midwives who graciously assisted in data collection.

Dr. Dori Pelz-Sherman, for her incredible gift for encouragement and constructive criticism.

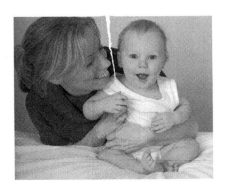

CHAPTER 1

The Importance
of Patterns

When I was a little girl, often my mother and grandmother would set up a large wooden quilting frame in the living room. The frame itself would be suspended from hooks in the ceiling, and a quilt would be stretched over the frame. Often several women would gather around, stitching the finished quilt top to layers of batting and backing. The quilt top itself was made up of fabric pieces cut into shapes and then sewn together in intricate patterns—Log Cabin, Sunbonnet Sue, Trip around the World, and Wedding Ring. These are some of the names given to the traditional patterns. The fabric for these beautifully designed and constructed quilt tops came from available fabric; it was not bought new in fat quarters at the craft store. To this day, I can still point out pieces of fabric sewn into these quilts and remember where they came from—my mother's dress, my grandmother's housecoat, my blouse, my nightgown, or my father's shirt.

Quilts can be a metaphor for the way we experience our lives. We remember the past, but not as a photograph or a recording. Our memories are more like artist's renderings of the past. Like the quilter who picks and chooses the part of the garment that will be included in a quilt block, cutting away the rest, we select what we consider to be the important parts of an experience and disregard or discount the rest (e.g., Conway, 2005).

One traditional quilt pattern is known as Tumbling Blocks. The skilled quilter assembles the light and dark fabrics of this pattern in a way that gives a three-dimensional look to the quilt top. If the quilter makes a mistake—say, the lights and darks are reversed in one of the blocks—it would catch our eye very quickly, because visually, we expect the regularity in this repeating pattern.

People are very good at recognizing patterns. Patterns may be expressed in space, such as letters on a page, chairs in rows, or bricks in a wall. Patterns may also be expressed in time, like musical rhythms, class schedules, seasons of the year, or family traditions transcending generations. Pattern recognition enables us to make sense out of the world, to predict what is going to happen based on what has already happened, and to exert some level of control over our lives and our destinies (Scheber, 2011). Pattern recognition is truly a wonderful capacity.

George Kelly (1963) first observed that forming mental patterns help us understand the world. We take all of our experiences, things we think and observe, and things that happen to us, and form a framework that helps us understand future events. Psychologists call this constructing our experience.

The psychology of personal constructs is a framework that explains how our past colors our present experiences. We're going to see that the way we look at the world is especially relevant when we talk about postpartum depression.

Seeing the World through Our Experiences

Beginning in infancy, we develop habits that helps us make sense of the world. This is a result of our ability to compare the present moment to past situations and to recognize repeating patterns (Scheber, 2011). We do not have to constantly relearn what to expect from familiar situations, nor do we have to constantly reinvent our responses. We are consciously aware of very little of this habitual pattern recognition. Most of the time, it just hums in the background, informing the way we think, feel, and behave without much fuss (Toomey & Ecker, 2007). We can be so preoccupied with a pressing problem that we are only vaguely aware of driving home from work, yet we are able to stop at red lights, make the correct turns, and brake for pedestrians. Once we have acquired a skill, our need to pay so much attention to it decreases. Reading this page is a good example. If you are a skilled reader, you are not sounding out the words, but are instead attending to the meaning of the words.

I have made a few quilts in my time, but my skills are not automatic and I must give quilting my undivided attention. My grandmother, by contrast, could quilt, carry on a conversation, and cook entire meals at the same time. Her quilting skills were automatic.

We also experience the world through our innate capacity to create, recognize, and participate in repeating patterns brought to us through our senses. That experience results in learning, a change in our behavior including voluntary movements, thoughts, feelings, and physiological reactions (De Houwer, Barnes-Holmes, & Moors, 2013). Learning is stored in memory for our future use. With enough experience, we do not have to pay attention, or be consciously aware, of the pattern to respond to it. Our behavior becomes automatic (Wigley, 2007).

Automatic behavior is crucial for our survival in a challenging world. If we had to pay total attention to every tiny decision we make every day, such as how to fold a t-shirt or how to change the television channel, there would not be enough attention left over to learn anything new or to consider the meaning of events (Feldon, 2007).

Similarly, there is just too much going on at any given moment for us to remember every tiny particle of information available to our senses (McWilliams, 2013). As I type this, my office environment is relatively quiet and dim. However, even in this relatively calm and well-known space, if I close my eyes, I can only remember parts of my own office. If I could remember it perfectly, as if I possessed an inner photograph, why would I need to search for the paperclips or wonder if I have a hairbrush around here somewhere? I attend to what I think is important and discard the rest.

It is important to note that I said I attend to what I think is important. This is a vital point because in picking and choosing the aspects of our inner and outer world that we will learn from and then store in memory, we make value judgments. If everything is important, then nothing is important. We instinctively know that and so we make choices about what we are going to pay attention to and what we judge to be significant (Lebreton, Jorge, Michel, Thirion, & Pessiglione, 2009). We don't just recognize patterns; we also create them (Toomey & Ecker, 2007).

Why Patterns Are Important in Depression

There's a now classic study that laid the foundation for much of our present understanding of depression. You might be familiar with it. Two researchers, who were studying learning in dogs, were trying to prime the dogs to learn faster. They put a dog in a wooden box that was wired to give electric shocks on one side. The box had two compartments separated by a door. At first, the researchers left the door open and the dog quickly learned to jump through the door to the other side, escaping the shock. Then the researchers locked the door, thinking that the dogs would respond faster when the door was opened next trial. Surprise! When they exposed the dogs to a mild shock without an escape option, once the door was opened, the dogs did not try to escape. They had learned that there was no escape and they had quit trying to find one. This phenomenon was observed many times. It was named "learned helplessness" and, when extended to people, became a key element in our understanding of human depression (Seligman & Maier, 1967). People who find themselves in inescapable stressful situations also begin to shut down, and to get depressed (Kramer, Helmes, Seelig, Fuchs, & Bengel, 2014).

The dogs in this now-famous experiment recognized the pattern: shock without the possibility of escape or relief. When they were faced with an escape option, they discounted it. It was not a part of the pattern. In a sense, their suffering was part of their belief system. They were trapped by their belief in the inescapability of their predicament. They demonstrated for us a fundamental life principle: *It's not what happens to you, it's what you believe about it* (Joormann & D'Avanzato, 2010).

Similarly, we people can become trapped in the inescapable stress of a dysfunctional belief system. What may have begun as simple recognition of patterns in our childhood experiences can become self-perpetuating prisons in which we only see what makes sense to us, aspects of each and every situation that conforms to what we already expected. Our past is carried forward into the future through expectancies; we notice, remember, and ultimately respond to cues that conform to what we were expecting (Tambling, 2012).

Your expectancies drive the way you respond to other people as well as the physical environment (McCullough et al., 2011). First, you notice similarities that the present moment has to your past experiences. This sparks an emotional reaction, which in turn influences what you say, don't say, do, or don't do. Then the other person responds. Their response ultimately is either discounted as irrelevant or incorporated into your understanding of others. It is also incorporated into your understanding of yourself (Sedikides & Green, 2004). For example, if you have untrustworthy people and broken relationships in your past, you may anxiously watch others for signs of dishonesty, or you may feel more comfortable in relationships that repeat the old patterns, or both (Messman-Moore & Coates, 2007). This reflects expectancies that others behave dishonestly (expectancies of others) and that you are the kind of person that people lie to (expectancies of yourself). You know where you fit in these painful patterns, and if your expectancies are fulfilled, you have a sense of some control over your world.

Double Binds: When Patterns Collide

Humans can be remarkably inconsistent, especially with themselves. When these inconsistencies go underground as habitual patterns, people can wind up in situations where there are no acceptable moves to make (Gilbert & Gilbert, 2003). For example, a woman may strongly believe in pleasing others at all costs. What happens when pleasing one person means displeasing another? What happens when pleasing someone else is clearly destructive? What happens when others are clearly being unreasonable, and she becomes weary of turning backflips to please them? Along the same lines, how is the conflict resolved between believing it is critical to be successful and also believing that it is critical to avoid outshining others?

Known as double-binds, these conflicting beliefs ultimately lead to an internal stalemate, when neither making a decision nor failing to make a decision will help. There is no way, within the existing belief system, to become unstuck and to resolve the dilemma. There is a sense of being "damned if I do, and damned if I don't." In the face of such a conundrum, an emotional and motivational shutdown occurs. This is depression (Gilbert & Gilbert, 2003).

The good news is that we can change our beliefs. When we recognize the underlying patterns that we have overlearned and relied upon, perhaps from earliest childhood, a process known as "insight," then we can make conscious choices about them (Levitt et al., 2004). Insight allows us to evaluate and change our beliefs and expectations about ourselves and the world. The work involved in gaining and making use of insight, especially regarding the beliefs and expectations that put us in those nasty double-binds, may be gradual and slow, but the pay-off is enormous.

The Two Hits of Depression

In order to experience an episode of depression, there must be "two hits," so to speak (Worlein, 2014). The first hit is personal vulnerability to getting depressed. What makes you vulnerable? It can be that you believe the negative things people say to you or you may be trying to please everyone, which puts you in a double-bind. The second hit for depression is life stress. If you are already vulnerable, and you experience significant stress, you are at higher risk for getting depressed (Hammen, 2005).

No matter how stressful pregnancy and postpartum have been, that first hit of depression vulnerability is needed for depression to develop in the postpartum period (Hammen, 2005). Postpartum depression is more likely if the stress of this period coincides with sensitive areas of life that already generate a sense of helplessness and inadequacy (Hammen, 2005). For example, if family relationships are not great, the stress of having a new baby may lead to depression. After all, the baby is a brand-new family member and represents a new family relationship.

No matter how planned the pregnancy was, no matter how closely the labor and delivery corresponded to the birth plan, and no matter how healthy and easy the baby is, the process of having a baby is stressful.

The stress is multiplied when there are also factors such as:
- *the pregnancy was unplanned,*
- *there was an unexpected need for pain medication, a c-section, or a labor induction,*
- *the baby is sick, premature, or colicky,*
- *you don't have anyone to help you, or*
- *you have a history of trauma or abuse.*

There are other areas that are relevant as well, such as a new mother's level of confidence in her own ability to be responsible and care for a helpless infant, her marital security, her sense of financial or material stability, and confidence in her ability to juggle the challenges of career and the mother role (Hammen, 2005).

The point of exploring these possibilities is to help new mothers recognize that underlying beliefs about important areas of life are tightly related to becoming depressed. The good news is that each woman's belief system was constructed by her, for her. Because of this liberating truth, each woman has the power to deconstruct and reconstruct what she believes. In other words, each new mother holds her own keys to recovery from postpartum depression.

The Basis of This Book

This book is based on research conducted with real women attending their postpartum obstetrical check-ups. These new mothers answered questions about their depression symptoms, their attitudes toward themselves as mothers as well as toward their infants, and their belief systems about other people and interpersonal relationships. The answers gathered from asking these questions made it clear that the symptoms of postpartum depression are associated with problematic beliefs about self and others, and are also associated with less adaptive beliefs about motherhood and the baby. Our results allowed us to construct a model that explains how early experiences contribute to depression symptoms during the postpartum period:

- Experiences of criticism and rejection in relationships are encoded into the personal construct system as a certain kind of perfectionism known as socially prescribed perfectionism, in which women have a deep-seated belief that important others expect perfection (or at least, others expect more than they have to give). Because life itself gives everyone abundant evidence that they are not perfect, believing that important others expect perfection puts women in a perpetual no-win situation.

- These critical and rejecting experiences also lead to deeply and preferentially taking the imagined viewpoint of others when thinking about the self. One's own point of view is secondary to what others may be thinking. This also puts women in a no-win situation, because one's own point of view still exists, and exists for a reason, despite being constantly subjugated to "what do others think?"

> ### Beliefs That Can Lead to Postpartum Depression
>
> - *Feeling like you need to be perfect.*
>
> - *Feeling that your point of view is secondary to everyone else's.*
>
> - *Feeling that your needs are always secondary to the needs of others.*
>
> - *Self-silencing and not sharing how you really feel.*

- Preferentially taking others' presumed viewpoint, and at the same time believing that others expect too much, leads to distressing ways of being in intimate relationships. These ways of being include self-silencing (squelching parts of one's self in an effort to preserve a relationship) and believing that to care for someone means to always subjugate personal needs to those of the other person. These ways of being in a relationship lead to a pervasive feeling of being a different person on the inside than what is displayed to others. The distressing beliefs about others' expectations and about what is required to maintain intimate relationships are seldom challenged because important parts of the real self are kept quiet, and therefore, there is little opportunity for these beliefs to be tested and revised.

- When a woman with such distressing beliefs about relationships becomes a mother, her beliefs about herself-in-relationship tend to be transferred over to her relationship with her baby. She tends toward rigidly high expectations of herself as a mother and negativity toward the mother role.

- The end result of this process is higher levels of depression symptoms in the postpartum period (Thompson & Bendell, 2014).

This book is designed to explain the social and cognitive processes leading to postpartum depression, and to give depressed new mothers insight and support to help themselves. It is also intended to aid professionals that care for new mothers, such as physicians, midwives, and therapists. Body and mind work together, so while medical treatments like antidepressant medications target the healing of the body, so we must also consider personal and social change that targets the healing of the mind.

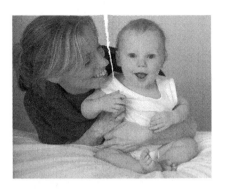

CHAPTER 2

The Signs and Significance of Postpartum Depression

My husband was in his fourth year of medical school when we found out I was pregnant for the first time. I had recently quit a highly stressful full-time job, so instead of seeking a new full-time position during pregnancy, I went to work for a temp agency. This augmented the stipend my husband got from the U.S. Air Force for his health professions' scholarship. Despite the money woes inherent in our life situation, we decided that after the baby was born, I would stay at home full time.

From an obstetrical standpoint, the pregnancy was uneventful. During my first trimester, my husband completed a six-week family practice rotation in northern California and I accompanied him. This experience might have been an adventure if it had not been marked for me by increasing anxiety. After returning home to Dallas, I became anxious about navigating Dallas traffic, and eventually turned down any temp jobs that required me to drive across the metroplex.

It did not occur to me that I did not have to suffer from this crippling anxiety. It was part of my pattern and it seemed normal to me. I was having a baby. I had no money. My husband was always busy, swept along by the Niagara Falls of medical school. I liked planning and security, but my plan seemed to be leading me away from security. Anxiety was so automatic that I didn't even give it a name.

My labor began vaguely one evening with contractions that were regular but not painful. I spent a restless night wondering if this was real labor or more Braxton-Hicks contractions. The next morning, I went to labor and delivery where my labor was confirmed. By about 10:00 a.m., I had to be put on a pitocin drip, and soon afterward received epidural pain relief. Our first son was born at 5:50 p.m. Delivery was vaginal, but accompanied by fourth-degree perineal tears. I remember vividly the contrast between mine and my husband's reaction to our newborn son. He was blissfully excited and moved to tears; I was exhausted and numb, thinking blankly, "Oh. It's a baby. Fancy that." I was drained physically and vastly underconfident in my ability to take care of this frighteningly tiny human being. In retrospect, it is fortunate that I had decided to breastfeed. This turned out to be something I could do, and something nobody could do for me. I'm not sure I would have touched my son in those first few days if not for the breastfeeding. I was so unsure of myself.

In many senses, neither my husband nor I had adequately separated from our families of origin, a situation that became sadly apparent in the hours and days following our son's birth. Both families showed up, and pressure began to build for both of us to please, to do things "right," and to make both sets of relatives happy. We needed both emotional and practical support, but often there seemed to be more drama than support going on. His brother was getting married across the state in three weeks, and he felt pressure from his family to bring the baby and me along, a pressure he passed along to me. My family strenuously objected to this plan. I was exhausted, physically injured, and overwhelmed. I also had no idea what I really wanted or how to say a firm and calm "no" to anyone. Instead, I did a lot of crying, arguing, and exploding. I quickly descended into depression. I remember one day during those first few postpartum weeks, sitting in the bathtub and wishing I could die.

It was only after years had passed, and public understanding of postpartum depression increased, that it occurred to me that I had experienced postpartum depression. I consider myself both fortunate and unfortunate. I was fortunate in that I never became actively suicidal, but unfortunate in that I didn't know enough to ask for help, and that there was no one there to recognize that I was in trouble. I was college educated. I was middle-class. I was married and my husband was a medical student who eventually became an obstetrician himself. I had even had a prior episode of depression in college. Yet, I still went without diagnosis and without treatment.

I believe that I had a depressive episode after the birth of each of our sons, and also during the prolonged and stressful international adoption process for our daughter. As time went on, the onset of a depressive episode morphed from primarily

emotional symptoms to primarily physical ones. A classi-
cally depressed mood was replaced by numbness and brain
fog. Sleeping too much was replaced by awakening at three
o'clock in the morning and being unable to go back to sleep.
Hopeless thoughts and feelings of being stuck were replaced
by overwhelming exhaustion. There came a time for me when
even thoughts of death were indulgences I could not afford. I
had a family, a home, and responsibilities. I had children who
needed me. Unfortunately, there were long periods where they
just got the bare minimum because I was ill and I didn't even
know it. Somewhere in my bones, though, I felt it keenly.

Postpartum depression, by definition, is a depressive episode that occurs after the birth of a baby. Because you have to experience depressive symptoms for at least two weeks to be diagnosed with depression, technically any depressive episode with a postpartum onset can't be diagnosed before two weeks postpartum (American Psychiatric Association, 2013). However, considering that many women diagnosed with postpartum depression were already depressed during pregnancy, some mothers, in reality, may be depressed from the start (Eberhard-Gran, Tambs, Opjordsmoen, Skrondal, & Eskild, 2004). Estimates are that between 10% and 25% of all postpartum mothers experience depression (e.g., Appolonio & Fingerhut, 2008; Centers for Disease Control and Prevention, 2008; Gausia, Fisher, Ali, & Oosthuizer, 2009). The wide range in these estimates reflect the different depression rates according to your ethnicity and how long after childbirth an episode is labelled "postpartum" (e.g., Bina, 2008). Sometimes any depressive episode during the baby's first year is called "postpartum," but Kendall-Tackett prefers the term "depression in new mothers," since it can occur anytime in the first year and "postpartum" becomes a bit of a misnomer (Kendall-Tackett, 2010). At any rate, it is clear that postpartum depression is a common occurrence. You are not alone.

The difference between a challenging life circumstance and a stressful one lies in our perceptions. A challenging life circumstance is one that we recognize may be difficult but lies fully within our capacity to overcome. A stressful life circumstance is one that we recognize is difficult and harbor doubt that we can deal with it. The more of a gap between the level of challenge and our perceived ability to cope, the more stress we experience (Johnson & Johnson, 2010). Most risk factors for postpartum depression are directly or indirectly tied to stress.

For example, if you are a teenager when you have your baby, you are more likely to get depressed (Carlson, 2011). Teens usually have more challenges when they become mothers, such as changes in their future plans, difficulty finishing school, the high cost of raising a child, more dependence on their own parents at a time when they were gaining more independence, and complications with the relationship with the baby's father.

Being an older mother can put you at higher risk for depression as well (Carlson, 2011). Older moms may have already been through multiple infertility treatments and may be very conscious of the potential for their baby to have health problems, or they may have older children and may have not been expecting to be pregnant again. They may feel out-of-sync with women their own age and other new moms, with different career concerns and more aches and pains, or even more serious health concerns, while pregnant.

Other things that put women at greater risk of postpartum depression are a history of trauma or abuse, a bad marriage (Zelkowitz et al., 2008), especially one that includes violence (Dennis & Vigod, 2013); living in poverty; being a single mom (Brett, Barfield, & Williams, 2008), and having a difficult pregnancy or difficult labor and delivery (Sorenson & Tschetter, 2010). Although, it is important to remember that the fundamental principle of depression is *it's not what happens to you, it's what you believe about it,* women with any of these risk factors are especially vulnerable when faced with the challenges of the postpartum period.

Signs of Postpartum Depression

Depressive symptoms are illness behaviors (Yirmiya et al., 2000) and are a way to cope with stressful relationships and critical inner voices (Kanter, Busch, Weeks, & Landes, 2008). They lead you to withdraw from others, to seek rest and quiet, and to avoid taking on responsibilities. The withdrawal from pressure, stress, and difficult relationships may feel like a relief initially; however, these illness behaviors are not helpful in the long run. Even in the short run, depressive behaviors, such as staying in bed or in the house, neglecting personal hygiene, and abandoning enjoyable or fulfilling activities prolongs and exacerbates depression (Veale, 2008).

Postpartum depression is not just about feeling blue or having a low mood, although that must be present to call it depression. Other symptoms are bone-sucking fatigue, sleep disturbances, over- or under-eating, noticeable physical restlessness or sluggishness, diminished pleasure or enjoyment in life, overblown guilt feelings, thoughts of death, and brain fog. A depression diagnosis requires at least five of these symptoms, but with such a long list of potential symptoms, any two depressed women can have very different experiences. Depression and its various symptoms can also vary in severity, from mildly annoying to completely debilitating. For a depressive episode to quality for a diagnosis of major depressive disorder, however, symptoms do need to be severe enough to impair your daily life or cause you significant distress (American Psychiatric Association, 2013).

Other experiences associated with depression include: poor motivation; feeling pain more intensely, including flu-like aches and pains, headaches, back aches, and joint pain; emotional numbing rather than feeling low or blue; fragmented sleep, especially early-morning awakening; vivid nightmares or anxiety dreams; irritability, impatience and low tolerance for others or for minor setbacks; pessimism and negativity; hopelessness or feeling as if nothing will ever be OK again; inability to get excited or anticipate anything; indecisiveness; nervousness or feeling anxious and keyed up; and, feeling overwhelmed and inadequate even to do routine tasks (e.g., Wise, Fishbain, & Holder-Perkins, 2007).

Sometimes people think that having a low mood just means sadness. However, sadness is not the only emotion associated with a low mood. A mood is an emotional state that stays with you over time, rather than a quick and fleeting reaction that comes in response to a particular situation. A low mood may be experienced as not being able to get motivated, excited, or energized about much over a long period of time; it may be experienced as not feeling much at all, as if happiness, joy, sadness, anger, and fear are completely gone. Irritability may also be the most prominent sign of a low mood, because you feel unable to handle minor hassles or setbacks.Sometimes depression can feel as if you just don't have the resources that it takes to do what you need to do. It feels as though you cannot face the day. You are drained, exhausted, and overwhelmed all the time. This is the global feeling of depression. All the individual symptoms combine to create this global sense of depletion and defeat.

Postpartum Depression = Plain Old Depression

The symptoms and experience of postpartum depression are indistinguishable from depression in other life periods. As a disorder that can manifest with a widely variable symptom profile, there is no particular symptom unique to postpartum depression and no symptom profile that sets a postpartum episode apart (American Psychiatric Association, 2013). However, the unique challenges of the postpartum period can make it hard to distinguish depression from normal adjustment to new motherhood. New mothers are typically tired, from the physical challenges of labor and delivery and from disturbed sleep due to having a newborn to care for. This normal fatigue can cause a new mother to be short-tempered or weepy, and can interfere with her ability to concentrate. Also, having a baby is normally associated with weight change and other bodily adjustments, which can mask some of the other physical symptoms of depression. It is important that professionals charged with diagnosing postpartum depression take the time to sort out the differences between the normal challenges of the postpartum period and depression symptoms (O'Hara & McCabe, 2013).

Depression Symptoms: Survival of the Fittest?

Generally speaking, inherited traits that make an organism less fit and healthy have a tendency to die out in just a few generations (Raison, Jain, Maletic, & Draud, 2009). Therefore, it is somewhat of a conundrum that depression, a debilitating and recurring illness that tends to run in families, and is thought to be at least partly biologically based, has not only remained a part of the human legacy, but appears to be becoming more and more prevalent. The first clue to this seeming conundrum is that depression is associated with increased levels of pro-inflammatory molecules produced by the immune system (Kendall-Tackett, 2007). There is even some evidence that depressed people run low-grade fevers, as if depression is a febrile illness. When a person is experiencing symptoms of depression, there is a corresponding increase in inflammation throughout the central nervous system. Additionally, although specific depression genes have not been definitely identified, it does appear that the best candidates are also associated with heightened immune response and heightened production of inflammation in response to pathogens (Raison & Miller, 2013).

Throughout human history, the biggest threat to survival has been infectious disease. The humans with the most robust capability of fighting off infection were the ones that would survive. In environments of high pathogen (germ) load, running high on inflammation would confer a survival advantage. This theory is supported by findings that in areas of the world without reliable clean water and modern sanitation standards, the proportion of older people with the high inflammation variants of certain genes is much greater than in areas with reliable clean water and sanitation. In other words, people with high inflammation versions of these genes are much more likely to survive into old age when the environmental germ load is high (Raison & Miller, 2013).

Those in the developed world, who can generally expect clean water, minimal exposure to sewage, and other advantages that minimize infection risk, experience the flip side of high inflammation levels: the chronic diseases of aging, such as Type II diabetes, heart disease, and some types of dementia. A depressive response to stress may also fall into the category of the down side of having a vigorous inflammatory response (Raison & Miller, 2013).

The Depressed Woman

It is important to note that women get depressed much more often than men. This gender difference begins in early adolescence and continues into old age (e.g., Leach, Christensen, MacKinnon, Windsor, & Butterworth, 2008). So, if depression can be biologically explained as a down side to a vigorous inflammatory response, why do women suffer from it so much more often than men? The explanation may lie at the intersection of biology, psychology, and culture.

Immerman and Mackey (2003) have provided a theoretical framework for understanding the way social relationships and physiology have interacted to encourage the surviving and thriving of female depression. Stretching back into prehistory, males and females have survived to pass on their DNA by being interdependent on one another. Typically, the woman would agree to be sexually faithful to one partner, thereby insuring that her children were also his children. The man would agree in exchange to protect and to provide for the woman and her offspring. If the woman broke this agreement, the man could simply abandon her and her children. If the man broke the agreement, however, a woman was relatively stuck. In a hostile environment in which survival was never assured, packing up the kids and leaving was probably seldom an option. In these situations, a woman had no good options: the very definition of a double-bind. In this sort of situation, depression might have served an important function. If a woman began to manifest depressive symptoms, such as fatigue, fragmented sleep, agitation, sluggishness, and low motivation, it would cause a hardship for the entire clan. Other symptoms, like weepiness, low mood, feelings of guilt, negativity, or suicidal gestures would make it obvious that the problem was with her family situation. The man's family and friends, probably the ones who had to take over when the woman's productivity went down, might exert social pressure on him to get his act together. In this way, female depression may have increased the chance that a mate would be pressured to perform his agreed-upon function as protector and provider. Depression-prone women may have therefore survived in greater numbers to pass their DNA along to contemporary women (Immerman & Mackey, 2003).

Depression as an Adaptation

Although, it may seem at first glance that the "inflammatory" and the "social contract" explanations are incompatible, remember that the inflammatory response is primarily to enable us to fight off pathogens, or physical germs. It really is quite extraordinary that our nervous systems can interpret psychological or emotional stressors as invaders that require an immune response. These two explanations can fit together in this way: women whose bodies were able to recognize psychological stress, especially those nasty double-bind situations, as requiring an inflammatory immune response may have survived in greater numbers. As we know that interpersonal and social stress in particular can lead to depression, it is as if our bodies and brains respond to toxic relationships and ways of interacting with others as if they are germs to be fought off. If we don't practice healthy ways of being with others, our physical bodies will throw up high levels of inflammation in an attempt to protect us.

Putting It All Together

Of course, men can get depressed too, so depression is certainly not a female-only disorder (e.g., Kendler, Gardner, & Prescott, 2006). As discussed previously, any time people find themselves in double-binds or no-win situations, they may get depressed. However, over many millennia societal and cultural processes may have put women in double-binds more often. This may have been a social environment that, like geographical areas without clean water or modern sanitation, favored those with a vigorous inflammatory response.

The postpartum period brings together many different elements that may be stressful to the depression-vulnerable woman. Your body needs to heal from labor and delivery. Your life has been disrupted first by pregnancy and then by a newborn. Your partner may also be struggling with this huge life change, and your relationship may need to adjust to your new reality. Often one or both new grandmothers spend some time helping out during the postpartum period, with varying degrees of actual helpfulness. Other family members are likely to visit. Job and career concerns may be on your mind as well. It is a time that may activate some of those double-binds in your belief system that are otherwise somewhat dormant.

We cannot go back and change our genetic inheritance or our evolutionary history. The conflicting expectations of women, particularly mothers, that our culture or subculture imposes is pretty much out of our control as well. What we can do, instead, is to make different choices for ourselves, in the interest of combatting and recovering from depression.

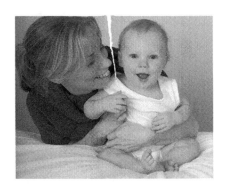

CHAPTER 3

It's Not Me, It's Us: Relational Roots of Postpartum Depression

In the past few years, I began to use social media. Social media is a great tool to stay connected to people across time and space. I have also made the observation that my social media networks act as schematics of my relationships stretching back to my childhood. Scrolling through my lists of connections, I have considered the quality of relationships I have had with people over my lifetime. This sort of life relationship review can be very powerful for women who struggle with depression. Whether you are experiencing depression for the first time during the postpartum period, or whether you have experienced multiple depressive episodes at different periods in your life, the information you gain about yourself can be illuminating.

The idea of a relationship life review came to me when patterns almost came leaping off the screen at me. Earlier in life, the closer the friendship supposedly was, the more likely it was that the relationship was marked by me being more interested in them than they were in me. Sometimes, the other person was domineering and bossy. Sometimes, the other person treated me as an afterthought, or someone to be with if nobody else was available. I was most comfortable with someone who kept me at arm's length, and who retained all or most of the power in the relationship.

On the other hand, I didn't really know what to do with a person who didn't operate on this principle of skewed relationship power. I never put a lot of effort into those relationships. During my review, it was with a little shock that I realized that if someone treated me as if I were valued, I reacted emotionally as if there was something wrong with them. I kept them at arm's length.

These kinds of patterns are not necessarily global across all areas or periods of life. My own relationship review turned up some healthy relationships as well as unhealthy ones, and the healthy pattern has strengthened and solidified over time. However, the unhealthy pattern was widespread enough that, especially early on, I was subjected to frequent subtle rejection. I also missed out on the joy of being close to some really lovely people.

This chapter focuses on patterns having to do with your relationship with yourself and others, and how those patterns relate to depression. In some cases, the research literature has only identified these patterns in people who are actually depressed. In other cases, these patterns have been identified in people who are at risk for depression. This fine distinction will not be made here. What really matters is, if you are struggling with postpartum depression, whether you identify with any of these patterns.

While toxic relationship patterns do not yield easily, it is possible to change them. It is worth the struggle. Any draw you feel to rejecting relationships can diminish and eventually dissipate. New patterns are established one relationship at a time, as mutual respect and support are built thoughtfully and intentionally. When others are distant or hostile, you may hear the internal whisper, "try harder," but as recovery progresses, another voice begins to whisper back, "accept what they are telling you." Relationships began to be viewed in a more balanced way; you begin to more clearly identify the role that the other person is playing in the relationship, and to more clearly define what is reasonable for you to do to keep the relationship afloat.

If a person is telegraphing stay away, or submit to me, a choice arises whether or not to continue to pour resources into the relationship. In many situations, this is virtually the only choice available for you to make. Sometimes, the wise thing to do is to walk away for a moment. When the problem is more entrenched, the wise thing may be to walk away for a season. Truly toxic relationships may require you, as an emotionally healthy adult, to walk away for a lifetime.

Human beings cannot do and be everything, so whenever you say "yes" to one thing, you are saying "no" to another. The first step in changing life patterns is recognizing to what you are saying "yes" and to what you are saying "no." It is then that change becomes possible.

Those who are prone to depression harbor unhealthy beliefs about themselves and others that lead to painful symptoms, as well as problem behaviors in relationships. Some examples of these unhealthy beliefs are:

- *I am defective.*
- *I am inadequate.*
- *I am incapable.*
- *Other people hold all the cards.*
- *Other people are untrustworthy.*
- *Other people will tell me what I want to hear, but they will stab me in the back.*
- *I do not have what it takes to inspire loyalty and commitment in others.*
- *I am a magnet for bottom-feeders who will use me and leave me.*
- *I do not deserve respect, loyalty, or love. I do not expect them from others.*

Depression Has a Social Nature

Depressed people have certain attitudes, traits, and behaviors that mark their relationships and interactions with other people. These characteristics tend to repel others, to damage relationships, and even to act as a contagion that passes depression on to others.

During the postpartum period, relationship stress will likely rear its ugly head. Often family members are coming to visit, to see the new baby and because new parents usually need some help from others. If family members are sources of depressive beliefs you harbor about people, then their appearance at this time in your life can be stressful. It also may be stressful to discover that the relationship with your partner must adjust and change to accommodate the needs of an infant and a different family structure. Even the new baby can be stressful for someone who expects relationships to be unsatisfying, painful, or difficult. This is a brand new person with whom to be in relationship.

It is an important part of the process to not only identify the belief system and underground patterns that contribute to depression, but also to identify possible sources of those patterns. Until you begin to do this important work, it will seem as if your beliefs about yourself, others, the world, and the future just fell from the sky, or were ordained by God or the universe. You will continue to accept your depressive beliefs as *The Inescapable Truth* about yourself.

Developing a theory of how you got to this point helps you step back and examine your beliefs critically. Critically examining your belief system should be distinguished from being critical of yourself or of others. The point of this examination is "what is" and "what was," not "what should have been." If the thought of identifying some sources of your depressive beliefs makes you uncomfortable or as if you might be adopting a victim mentality, rest assured that this is not about assigning blame. In many families, relationship patterns go back many generations, with each generation just repeating what they know from experience. This is as much of a reason as biology why depression tends to run in families (Hammen, Shih, & Brennan, 2004). Furthermore, these family patterns may have originated in extreme hardship, such as war, famine, grinding poverty, persecution, and other types of dire threat. Many of us do not have to look back very many generations to find ancestors who lived in conditions of lifelong hardship. Family patterns that are associated with depression may have evolved to help people survive in the ancestral environment (Belsky, 2011). The task, rather than assigning blame, is to recognize and understand the patterns and to make conscious choices about what to carry forward into the next generation.

Stepping back and realizing that your deeply entrenched depressive beliefs about yourself and others came from sources you can identify, and by extension, are not necessarily The Absolute Truth, is vitally important work. This work naturally leads to asking equally vital questions about those beliefs:

- *Is this true?*
- *How well is this working for me?*
- *Is investing in this belief of mine worth the depression or other negative consequences?*
- *What are the consequences of changing?*
- *Who says I have to be this, do this, or believe this?*
- *Who is the boss of me?*

The Importance of Relationships

People need each other. That need is as fundamental as our need for air, water, and food. People not only need others during the helplessness of infancy and the vulnerability of childhood, but we need others throughout the lifespan. People also need to be needed by others! At the most primal level, huddling together with other people increases our chances for survival. Weather, famine, disease, wild animal attacks, and accidental injury were constant threats to early human ancestors and are still problems contemporary societies must manage (MacDonald & Jensen-Campbell, 2011).

Human babies are some of the most vulnerable creatures on earth. Being left alone during infancy spells certain death. The time we spend between birth and adulthood is protracted, which allows our bodies and brains to develop slowly and gives us the most sophisticated and complex behavioral range of any living species. This prolonged period of immaturity is beneficial in that it gives us the flexibility to adapt to many different environments. While instinctive behaviors in other animals allows them to survive and thrive in a specific environment, humans can live almost anywhere on earth (e.g., Julian, Wilson, & Moore, 2009).

We may not have instincts hardwired into our brains, but there are some kinds of environmental stimulation that the human brain is prepared to receive. When this kind of stimulation is available, the developing person responds to it with growth, learning, and behavior change. This is known as experience-expectant learning (Jones & Jefferson, 2011). It is crucial for healthy development to receive the expected experiences within the proper windows of time known as critical or sensitive periods (Hensch, 2004).

Perhaps the most fundamental experience that we are hardwired to expect is that of a stable, nurturing relationship with a loving caregiver, known as an "attachment relationship" (Sakaluk, 2013). Most often, this is the mother, since the mother carries the child inside her body and is equipped to nurse the baby at her breast. However, children can and do become strongly attached to fathers, grandparents, and others as well. When these important relationships are stable and nurturing, they can either supplement the mother-child bond or make up for what it lacks.

The absence of a stable and nurturing relationship during the critical period of infancy and toddlerhood leads to deficits in many areas of life, especially in the area of social learning and the ability to form meaningful relationships with others (McKenzie, Purvis, & Cross, 2014).

Most babies do have at least one person to whom they become attached, but the quality of these attachments varies. Every mother is different, with her own personality, physiology, spirituality, culture, and family background. Babies are all unique as well. As many as 14 different dimensions of infant temperament have been identified and measured (Costa & Figueiredo, 2011), meaning that even this early in life, the differences between people can be profound. However, there are some similarities observed across large groups of mothers and babies that help us understand how early attachment relationships are related to later experiences (Epkins & Heckler, 2011).

Studies of infants and their mothers have demonstrated that depression has a negative impact on the quality of the attachment relationship, on mother-baby interactions, on the child's development for several years after birth, and on the likelihood that the child will experience depression later in life (e.g., Goodman et al., 2011; Lefkovics, Baji, & Rigo, 2014). Babies of new mothers who were already depressed during pregnancy often have biological markers after birth, such as decreased vagal tone, greater activation in the right-frontal cortex of the brain, and skewed neurotransmitter profiles, that suggest that they are also depressed (Field, 2011). These are some of the important ways that depressive belief systems can be primed in young children, so that depression can be passed down for generations in families if the cycle is not interrupted.

People form and maintain attachment bonds with others throughout life. In adulthood, we are most likely to be bonded with another adult in a sexual or romantic relationship. Attachment bonds with our families of origin often persist throughout life as well, although they usually adapt and change. We form attachment bonds with our own children, and may even have close and long-lasting friendships that would qualify as attachment relationships. The quality of the bonds we form with others later in life is strongly related to the quality of our first attachment relationships, in which we learned on a very visceral level how to relate to significant other people (Galinha, Oishi, Pereira, Wirtz, & Esteves, 2014).

The Parenting Spectrum

With this fundamental understanding of the enormous impact that early relationships wield, taking a broad view of parenting styles will help to illuminate how these relationships either promote resilience or contribute to depression vulnerability. Recognizing and understanding the connections between childhood experiences and depression in adulthood, including postpartum depression, will support your recovery. It will also enable you as a new parent to make conscious choices about what parenting path to take with the next generation.

Emotionally Healthy Parenting

It is a universal challenge for parents to find a healthy balance between protecting a child from the very real dangers of this world and preparing that child to deal with the world independently.

Some parents seem to sail through this challenge, seamlessly transitioning through their child's many stages. Others stumble along the way, holding on too long or expecting too much, too soon. Parental protection lies on a continuum from extreme overprotection to extreme neglect, with desirable parenting occupying the middle ground somewhere in between (Iwaniec, Larkin, & McSherry, 2007). The trick to preparing a child adequately for life without overwhelming them is to keep their challenges within the level of difficulty that the child can master with their parent's help (Edwards, 2002).

Families who tend to have the best child outcomes are those who exert firm, consistent control over their children's behavior, and also consistently nurture a warm and loving relationship with their children. These families are aware of what can be reasonably expected according to the age, developmental level, intelligence, and abilities of each child (Overbeek, ten Have, Volleburgh, & de Graaf, 2007). These parents keep their expectations consistent and appropriate for each child.

Healthy parenting protects children from challenges they are not mature enough to face, and exposes children to developmentally appropriate opportunities to gain skill and competence (Edwards, 2002; Overbeek, ten Have, Volleburgh, & de Graff, 2007). Healthy parenting is thoughtful about when to lend a helping hand, and when to allow a child to fail. It should be noted that most parents fail at this particular challenge from time to time. Truly wise parents, realizing their mistakes, then have the opportunity to model learning from failure.

Disengaged Parenting

A neglectful parent is disengaged from the relationship and exposes the child to challenges, situations, and risks that the child is not prepared to face alone. These children are vulnerable to harm from a whole host of ills, including accidents, poor nutrition, sporadic school attendance, and human predators. If neglected children survive the very real dangers of inadequate parental supervision and protection, they may grow up feeling overwhelmed by the challenges of life, anxious that they are not equal to life's tasks, and overly vigilant to any hint of danger or risk. A neglected child may come to believe that she cannot win because the world is just too hard (Overbeek, ten

Have, Volleburgh, & de Graaf, 2007). If you were a neglected child, you may still carry a sense that the world is harsh and that you are not equal to its challenges (Wei & Kendall, 2014).

In less extreme cases, children may be taken care of physically but still experience emotional or psychological neglect. If your parents did not have a good sense of what children can handle emotionally at different stages, or if they were too fragile or caught up in their own problems, you may have been left to deal with hard emotional situations on your own.

When a child's successes, joys, problems, or concerns are met with indifference, lack of concern, ridicule, or other forms of insensitivity, the environment is *invalidating* (Yap, Allen, & Ladouceur, 2008). Invalidating environments dismiss or even punish a child when she tries to get emotional support for things that are important to her. Invalidating environments don't have to involve physical neglect or abuse. When to all appearances, it seems that your needs were taken care of, it can be challenging to acknowledge or understand that your emotional needs were invalidated. However, being raised in an emotionally invalidating environment leaves children with difficulty regulating, or coping effectively with their own emotions (Shenk & Fruzzetti, 2014). Depression can be understood as a type of problem with emotional regulation (Yap, Allen, & Ladouceur, 2008).

Overinvolved Parenting

If neglect is really bad, then overprotection must be really good, right? Not so. Although, overprotected children may be safer than neglected children from physical dangers, the psychological damage done to overprotected children can be severe (Epkins & Heckler, 2011). Trying too zealously to shield a child from failure or from all manner of risk can lead to a fragile child who wilts when faced with a challenge.

Parental overprotection sends the message that the world is an overwhelmingly scary and dangerous place that the child cannot survive without the parent's constant vigilance. Of course, this is true—in infancy. The truth of that statement, however, gradually decreases as the child grows toward adulthood. Overprotective parents are not keeping their child's challenges within an appropriate range any more than the neglectful ones. The message that overprotected children receive is that they are not competent, that they are helpless, that there is no escaping the parent's rigid control, and even if there was an escape option, it is far too scary to contemplate.

This, like the neglected child's belief that he or she cannot be successful because the world is too hard, is a kind of learned helplessness. Like the dogs exposed to a mild but uncontrollable shock, an overprotected child may come to believe that she cannot help herself and cannot function without the parent's guidance (Otani et al., 2013; Overbeek, ten Have, Volleburgh, & de Graaf, 2007). This goes against the goal of emotionally healthy parenting, which is to gradually prepare the child to live a full and mature adult life.

Emotional invalidation can also be a part of overprotecting families. The desire to individuate (or separate your identity) from your parents, and to gradually gain a measure of personal independence, is natural, healthy, and developmentally appropriate (Edwards, 2002). Families that discourage a child's appropriate expressions of individuality and personal agency are effectively invalidating important aspects of their child's emotional life (Barber, Xia, Olsen, McNeely, & Bose, 2012). Similar to the neglectful family environment, an overprotective environment in which the child's own perspective, opinions, and desires are routinely dismissed breeds depression vulnerability (Meites, Ingram, & Siegle, 2012).

Critical Parents

Those who are anxious about being accepted and approved of by other people are usually very, very sensitive to any signs of being rejected by others (McDonald et al., 2010). This doesn't appear out of nowhere. While some people may naturally be extra sensitive to negative feedback and may naturally react quickly and strongly to it (Gill & Warburton, 2012), there is usually some basis in real-world experience that creates this acute sensitivity to criticism and uncertainty about being accepted by others. Excessive criticism from parents, which is often part of depressed women's experience, can have this effect (Epkins & Heckler, 2011). Like other parts of your implicit belief system, once your alarm system begins to go off at the merest hint of criticism, it becomes resistant to change.

Underinvolvement with a child may lead a parent to callousness and lack of empathy. Overinvolvement with a child may lead to micromanaging the child. Either of these extreme parental positions may lead to excessive parental criticism. The neglectful parent criticizes because she is unable to empathize; the overprotective parent criticizes because she wants to shield the child from the consequences of making mistakes (Mills et al., 2007).

We cannot give what we do not possess. Parents who do not possess confidence and emotional maturity themselves will have a much harder time nurturing these qualities in their children. A parent who is critical and harsh may be preoccupied with personal problems or ignorant of what can be expected of a child at this developmental stage. She may be unable to imagine anyone else's perspective but her own, and may take childish mistakes or ignorance as a personal insult. These are some of the common roots of excessive parental criticism, and they originate inside the parent. Unfortunately, children do take it personally because they are not yet sophisticated enough to see beneath the surface (Lawson, 2000; Mills et al., 2007). Some parents may be unable to distinguish between the child and themselves emotionally. Whatever this type of parent dislikes about herself is punished in the child. She criticizes the child for not perfectly emulating the things about herself that she does like. She experiences her child's problems with the same distress that she experiences her own. The child is expected to perfectly reflect her own desires and goals. Misconduct, especially in front of others, is a personal insult. The parent does not have an adequate understanding that the child is not just an extension of herself. She believes her daughter either proves or disproves her own worthiness. When her daughter goes off-script, this type of parent experiences anxiety. This anxiety then produces accelerated controlling behavior, including harsh criticism (Lawson, 2000; Mills et al., 2007).

The Importance of Attachment Quality

We have examined parenting styles and the effects they have on children. Now it is time to take a look at parent-child attachment relationships, the way the quality of these relationships impact development, and how they may be passed from generation to generation. The quality of attachment relationships is a primary component of family life, and influences the other aspects of parenting. This exploration will help you understand how a parent's inner experience is transferred and transformed into the child's experience, and begin to point the way to healing.

Secure Attachment

Healthy attachments tend to promote adaptation and resilience even in the face of hardship. When these healthy attachments are absent or spotty, this adaptation and resilience becomes harder to come by (e.g., Perry, Sigal, Boucher, & Pare, 2006). Experience with attachment figures becomes embedded in our psyche early in life in the form of internal working models, which are well-developed systems of belief about ourselves in relationships with others (e.g., Johnson, Dweck, & Chen, 2007). Our underlying patterns of thought, feeling, and action flow from these internal working models, informing everything we do (e.g., Dimaggio et al., 2003).

The quality of the attachment relationship between baby and mother can be classified as either secure or insecure. As they grow and become more mobile, securely attached babies are emotionally free to explore their environment, discovering everything that babies are supposed to discover about the world. Secure babies check back with mother when they become distressed, but in general, they expect that the mother is present to keep them safe and will be there whenever she is needed. She is a comforting presence and a safe harbor as the baby explores the world. Fortunately, most babies appear to have secure attachment to at least one person (Bokhurst et al., 2003).

Insecure Attachment

Insecure babies don't have the same level of confidence that they have a safe harbor. An insecure-avoidant baby is disturbed about separation, but does not check in with her mother appropriately and shuts down emotionally in times of stress. Mothers of insecure-avoidant babies tend to be uncomfortable with the child's emotional neediness. These young children learn that the best way to keep the mother physically close is to suppress an indication of distress or need.

Children with insecure-avoidant attachment styles tend to develop patterns that keep others at a distance. These children begin coping at an early age with their mother's discomfort with closeness by keeping their natural needs for closeness turned off. Insecure-avoidant individuals continue to keep this system turned off by distraction, which manifests as inattention and hyperactive behavior in early childhood and as defiance and conduct problems later (Chen & Li, 2009; Sroufe, 2013). These behavior problems keep others at arm's length, which is the level of closeness within these individuals' comfort zone.

Insecure-anxious babies, by contrast, are clingy and anxious about any separation. They spend a lot of time and effort seeking contact with the mother and not enough time exploring and learning. Mothers of insecure-anxious babies tend to be unpredictable and only sporadically responsive to the child's needs. Sometimes such a mother is appropriately nurturing and sometimes not. The child learns to exaggerate signs of emotional neediness to get the mother's attention. Anxiously attached children will later tend towards internalizing problems, such as anxiety and depression. This is because they are excessively preoccupied with monitoring and controlling the mother's responses, which also requires a preoccupation with controlling and monitoring themselves. To control an attachment relationship requires you to stay one step ahead of the other person.

There are also some insecure babies that never develop reliable strategies to insure their own safety. Known as insecure-disorganized, these babies become confused and chaotic when stressed. These children

Earned Security of Attachment

When attachment security is examined in adults, it becomes apparent that there are some people who were insecurely attached in infancy and childhood, but who have one or more secure relationships in adulthood. These people are referred to as "earned-secure" and demonstrate that our history is not the sole determinant of our destiny (Saunders, Jacobovitz, Zaccagnino, Beuerung, & Hazen, 2011). We can change our relationship patterns.

usually have a mother who is either abusive or who has unresolved wounds from being abused herself. She may have periods in which she dissociates, becomes enraged and violent, or otherwise behaves in an extremely frightening manner. Later in childhood, these insecure-disorganized babies may gravitate to either an anxious or an avoidant coping style, or may fluctuate depending on many factors (Lecompte & Moss, 2014).

Gender Differences in Attachment Quality

Neither anxious nor avoidant attachment is truly specific to either gender. In infancy and toddlerhood, there have been no observed gender differences in the occurrence of either type of attachment insecurity. However, gender differences in attachment patterns do begin to emerge in middle childhood, with insecurely attached girls gravitating to the anxious type and boys to the avoidant type (Del Guidice & Belsky, 2010). It is relatively easy to see how these attachment patterns can be carried into adult life, causing relationship difficulties, such as the stereotypical "she wants more closeness, he wants more distance" pattern in troubled marriages. This emergence of gender differences during middle childhood suggests that the secure-insecure distinction is the primary way to understand attachment quality. Strategies for navigating close relationships may change according to factors, such as age, gender roles, and the emergence of new attachment figures, but it appears that the underlying security or insecurity usually remains stable (Del Guidice, 2008).

Anxiously Attached Girls

A pattern of intermittent or sporadic responding is one of the most powerful ways known to perpetuate a behavior. Effectively, if you are rewarded some, but not all, of the time, you will tend to try harder and harder until you do receive a response (Hogarth & Villeval, 2010). Anxiously attached girls are in relationship with others who intermittently respond to them, and so their preoccupation with getting other people's love and attention is sporadically rewarded with success. This keeps hope alive and the preoccupation with relationships going. The ways that anxiously attached girls try harder and harder over the years to insure that others are responsive to them becomes complex and deeply rooted in their ways of being in relationships. An anxiously attached girl begins to habitually view herself from the perspective of important others, overdeveloping her abilities to monitor herself and to conform to what she thinks others expect (Cutting & Dunn, 2002; Vliegen & Luyten, 2008). To stay one step ahead of others, she tries to anticipate what they are thinking and feeling, and to tailor her behavior to get what she needs and wants from them. Her own perspective becomes much less important than what others think or feel about her (Tan & Carfagnini, 2008). She may concentrate on seeking absolute merger with others to the exclusion of all other aspects of life, an impossible quest that leads to depression as hope of its success fails (Aube, 2008).

Self as an Object

Women with insecure attachment styles often develop a habitual way of stepping outside of themselves and, in the imagination, critically examining themselves from the perspectives of others. No life experience is completely entered into with abandon. Impression management becomes automatic, an overlearned response like riding a bicycle or signing her name. This way of self-perception from an external viewpoint develops very early and becomes a very fundamental part of the self. It is associated with the development of poor coping behaviors within intimate relationships. It is also associated with depression (Thompson & Bendell, 2014).

We live in a society where treating women and girls as objects is very common. When a woman or girl is objectified, she is not viewed by the other person as a human being with opinions, a mind, feelings, a soul, or even human rights. She is an object to be used. This can be seen in the phenomena of pornography, sex trafficking, and sexually based entertainment, such as strip clubs and topless bars. It can also be seen in the obsession our society has with a woman's external appearance and youthfulness, almost to the exclusion of any of her other attributes (Szymanski, Moffitt, & Carr, 2011).

We tend to accept treatment from others that is congruent with our beliefs about ourselves. Therefore, it may be that self-objectification sets women up to accept objectification from others. While there certainly may be many women who find themselves in the position of being objectified without having done it to themselves first, if self-objectification is her deeply ingrained way of being, it will seem more natural for her to accept others treating her as an object (Riva, Gaudio, & Dakanalis, 2014). We attract and accept treatment that we believe we deserve (Evraire, Ludmer, & Dozois, 2014).

No one can completely control the responses of others, including intimate relationship partners and close family members. Other people have their own experiences that drive the ways they respond. Relationships always involve at least two people and so are never completely within one person's control. When you feel completely responsible for a relationship that is only partially under your control, you will naturally have anxiety about it. You may become confused about what is and what is not your responsibility. Being stretched between two incompatible beliefs—I must and I can't— is a double-bind, and it is like being on a medieval torture rack. If you have an overdeveloped tendency to scrutinize yourself in an attempt to get what you need or want in a relationship, you are on this torture rack. Unless something happens to interrupt it, this intensive self-monitoring and self-criticism can be just effective enough to keep you doing it, over and over again, year after year, decade after decade, and relationship after relationship.

Conclusion

Everyone reading this had human parents, and that means that nobody had parents who were encouraging and supportive all the time. This is part of the human condition and what it means to be part of a human family. Your unique personal make-up, as well your experience besides your parents, contributes to how sensitive you are to criticism, how resilient to failure, and how much importance you put on positive or negative feedback. Even your experience with your parents might have a lot of variation. One of your parents may have been absent, critical, or perfectionistic, while the other may have been present, warm, and emotionally available. Life circumstances, such as divorce, bereavement, job loss, or the development of illnesses, may have put great stress on the family. In such cases, your experiences of the same parent may have differed over time. If you had good experiences with your grandparents, aunts, uncles, brothers, sisters, cousins, and even pets, and if you had the opportunity to forge bonds with friends, the effects of an inconsistent or frustrating parent may have been cushioned (e.g., Silverstein & Ruiz, 2006).

This chapter began with the importance of human relationships and has circled back to those nasty double-binds that are so associated with depression. If you have recognized some of your own experience in this discussion, you are likely becoming more aware of your habitual patterns of experiencing relationships. Now it is time to move on into how these patterns can manifest themselves in your adult relationships.

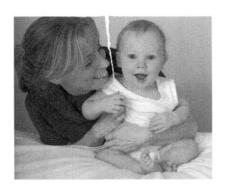

CHAPTER 4

Acting Depressed: Relationship Behaviors and the Perpetuation of Depression

When my husband was in first grade, a light bulb fell and shattered in the classroom. Six-year-old Doug took charge: "Everybody stand back. First we will pick up the big pieces, then we will sweep up the little ones" (Yes, he still is a take-charge kind of guy). He was recalling and making use of what he had heard at home about managing broken glass. What others have communicated to us with their own voices, we come to experience as a part of ourselves.

Most of us have had the experience of hearing our mother's voice in our thoughts. A college friend said that some time during her forties, she was at a dinner party in which a platter of fried chicken was passed. She wanted the biggest piece on the platter, but as she moved to take it, she heard her mother's voice, "Never take the biggest piece. Choose from one of the smaller pieces." She took a smaller piece. This happens on a more constant basis than most of us realize. The voices from our past may be loving, supportive, appreciative, and kind, or they may be harsh, critical, dismissing, demanding, and blaming. Either way, they are now incorporated into our experience of being ourselves.

There is a sense in which we are made up of community of voices, each voice representing a different aspect of ourselves and our experiences (Ribeiro et al., 2014). We have discussions and even arguments within ourselves as different voices come forward to contribute. Some voices dominate, other voices reciprocate, and still others are mostly silent until special circumstances cause them to speak. This is how we find ourselves in double-binds, as one voice says, "I must" and another voice responds "I can't" (Ribeiro et al., 2014).

Depression-prone people tend to get into relationships that create double-binds. People fit like locks and keys within important relationships. Therefore, a deep-seated sense that you don't deserve to be treated well will tend to attract people who are disrespectful or even worse. If you are consumed with self-doubt, you will tend to be drawn to those who are consumed with self-importance. Being in unsatisfying relationships with others can magnify the internal conflict between pursuing what feels good and right, and settling for what feels familiar. Choosing the unsatisfying familiar over relationship unknowns can create conditions of chronic stress in your life (Hammen, Shih, & Brennan, 2004).

People become comfortable with old patterns, even when they are painful. People seek confirmation of what they already believe about themselves, others, the future, and the world. The depressed have negative beliefs about themselves, and odd as it may seem, are most comfortable with people who confirm that negativity (Evraire, Ludmer, & Dozois, 2014). If you believe you are ugly, you will wonder what is wrong with someone who says you are beautiful. If you believe you are stupid, you question the intelligence of anyone who says otherwise.

We all seek a secure place from which to engage the world (e.g., Cassidy & Jones, 2014). If a warm and happy secure place is unavailable, you will choose a place that is merely stable rather than live in chaos.

Your life patterns, including a sense of what it means to be yourself, are formed through a lifetime of experience. The messages important people have sent you, and the interpretations you have put on those messages, are encoded into your body and brain. They are your secure place, your stable place within (Fivush, 2006). For those that expect it, negative feedback may be distasteful, but it is also paradoxically reassuring (Evraire & Dozois, 2011). It confirms your negative self-concept and bolsters the painful but stable place within.

Not understanding that they have placed both themselves and others in an impossible situation, depressed people persist in seeking reassurance. This reflects an effort to relieve inner pain (Evraire & Dozois, 2011). The more uncontrollable negative thoughts and perceptions feel, the greater the urgency for someone else to help. Unfortunately, if reassurances generally don't fit with your preexisting beliefs about your own defectiveness, any reassurances received are discounted. The search for more reassurance instead continues. This tends to drive others away, as constantly reassuring someone who won't be reassured is exhausting and frustrating.

People who have extensive experience with negative feedback typically continue to form and then persist in relationships with critical, negative people. An insatiable craving for reassurance works to erode positive relationships as well. Family members or friends can become drained and vulnerable to depression themselves (Dobson, Quigley, & Dozois, 2014).

The problem here should be obvious. While negativity may, at some level, affirm your sense of who you are, it is still negative. This double-bind consists of the conflict between the need for affirmation and the need for confirmation. A negative sense of self guarantees that having both is impossible. So depression leads to an internal dialogue that cancels out affirmation from others and to repetitive annoying behavior that drains beloved ones who want to help (Evraire & Dozois, 2011).

Manufacturing Stress

While stress happens to everyone, depression-prone people are better than most people at creating it. While this is not necessarily intentional, the habitual behaviors of depressed people tend to manufacture stress for themselves and others (Hankin, 2010). The depressed usually do not recognize the controllable nature of some of the stress they experience.

For example, harboring a sense that you are helpless or hopeless in important areas of life sparks behavior that makes stress worse. A major one of these behaviors is avoidance (Morris, Evans, Rao, & Garber, 2015; Ottenbreit, Dobson, & Quigley, 2014). Avoidance means attempting to cope by not coping. It leads to reluctance to commit to anything, putting off important responsibilities until the last minute, or failing to follow through. Avoidance creates a sense of impending doom, which is in itself stressful, and it can have dire consequences.

Sometimes depression-prone people can communicate a sense of entitlement, a "the world owes me a living" outlook. Outwardly, it may look as if the depressed think others are servants or that special favors are deserved. Inside, though, helplessness and hopelessness have stirred up frustration and anger, which may be expressed in demands for special treatment or caretaking (Newman, 2010). Seeking to turn over major responsibilities to others is another form of avoidance (Ottenbreitn et al., 2014). This, too, can have dire consequences.

Family, friends, and coworkers often share in the consequences when the depression-prone person avoids dreaded responsibilities or uncomfortable situations. Thus, avoidance drives a wedge in good relationships and intensifies anger, recrimination, and blame in poor ones. Some of the symptoms of depression, such as fatigue, poor motivation, diminished concentration, and oversleeping, may be understood as an involuntary type of avoidance (Ottenbreit et al., 2014). As relationships with others worsen and consequences for avoidance intensify, the depression-prone woman may retreat further and further into avoidance, whether in thought or deed.

Depression-prone people often have poor coping skills when it comes to managing life stress. If you tend toward depression, you may not have many stress-management tools to rely upon, even if otherwise, you are highly intelligent and very competent. You probably do not know how to stop the spiral downward when life begins to spin out of control. When anxiety and fear become crushing weights, someone who is depression-prone doesn't know how to make them stop (Ottenbreit et al., 2014).

Extreme Self-Sacrifice

A depression-prone woman often has a pattern of seeking connection with someone else to her own detriment (e.g., Tan & Carfagnini, 2008). While a drive for creating connections and community is a vital dimension of the healthy personality, some women tend to sacrifice too much in the quest for complete connection with someone else (O'Mahen, Flynn, & Nolen-Hoeksema, 2010). This someone else is usually, but not always, a romantic partner. Career goals; relationships with other family members, including one's own children; friendships; financial stability; personal strengths; and personal preferences may all be sacrificed in the pursuit of total connection with this other person.

There are many ways that seeking total connection with another can lead to a depressed state. The possibilities for double-binds are vast. A highly capable and intelligent career woman may experience intense conflict between her desires for personal success and independence, and her desires to merge into her partner's identity. A woman with few desires for career achievement may struggle to merge with an extremely busy or disengaged partner. A mother may attempt to live her life through her children, a Blackhawk-helicopter mom who is the despair of the kindergarten teacher, and eventually is the despair of her own offspring. Someday, if left unchecked, this drive to merge her identity with those of her children may stunt their launch into adulthood. Certainly, it will invite devastation and depletion when they leave her with an empty nest.

Even if you find someone willing to tolerate such an intense desire for merger, human relationships inevitably disappoint to some extent. Misunderstandings happen. Tempers flare. People find themselves out of sorts with one another. These little ruptures in relationships can loom large in your mind if you believe that all must be sacrificed on the altar of synchrony with someone else. Eventually, this belief, combined with the inevitable disappointments of human companionship, can lead to depression (Jin, Van Yperen, Sanderman, & Hagedoorn, 2010).

Little Miss Perfect?

While striving for excellence can be a source of joy and fulfillment, striving to be perfect can be a source of frustration and discouragement. This is because there really is no such thing as "perfect." There will always be another discovery to find, another invention to create, and another person who is just a little bit better. There will always be some way that you can improve upon your performance.

Perfectionism is at its most toxic in the form of socially prescribed

This is particularly true when it comes to mothering. Mothering is a highly individualized undertaking. What works for one family might be an epic failure with another. Yet, it seems as if women are all too eager to judge one another's mothering choices. Are you a stay-at-home mommy? You must be letting your brain stagnate and teaching your daughter harmful female stereotypes. Are you a career mommy? You must be neglecting your child and teaching your child she is not as important as your job. Living in an atmosphere of judgment, actual or perceived, usually results in one of two paths. Some women engage in frantic overzealous activity to prove their worthiness. Others drop out and quit trying. Some try a little of both.

perfectionism, or a deep sense that important other people expect perfection (Hill, Hall, & Appleton, 2011). This is especially true if you really want to please other people. You are likely very acutely and painfully aware of your own personal imperfections, which creates a double-bind of "I must be perfect" and "I can't be perfect" (Thompson & Bendell, 2014). If you want to please one person, then it is also likely you want to please several, or many, people. Even more double-binds arise when those people have conflicting expectations. It's no surprise that socially prescribed perfectionism is common in depression-prone women (e.g., Flett, Besser, Hewitt, & Davis, 2007).

A history of parental criticism and inconsistency, discussed in the previous chapter, can leave you feeling as if important other people expect too much, and that you can never be enough to satisfy (Enns, Cox, & Clara, 2002). If others expect perfection, and if you cannot be perfect, then you feel unworthy of respect, attention, love, and care. Perfectionistic demands from others may seem normal. You may believe that you are unworthy if you cannot figure out what is expected and fulfill those expectations perfectly. So you continually strive to be perfect, often becoming a high achiever. You were hoping success would make you happy, but instead, you suffer from intense anxiety. Or, perceiving that expecting perfection is unreasonable, you may give up and become a foot-dragger, procrastinator, and under-achiever (Ottenbreit et al., 2014). If this is you, then you think that if you can just delay trying, or if you have an excuse for not trying very hard, then maybe it won't hurt so much to fail (Steel, 2007).

Squelching Yourself

Often, women who are vulnerable to depression have trouble being totally genuine within close relationships. You may find yourself squelching important parts of who you are with your partner or your family because you fear rejection or abandonment (Flett et al., 2007). While it is sometimes prudent to carefully select the way you present yourself in public, to strangers, or in the workplace, if you can't express your true self in your closest relationships, the stress of keeping up the facade can become painful and difficult to bear (Flett et al., 2007).

Women who have trouble being completely real or genuine in close relationships silence their own voices. You self-silence when you habitually deny your personal needs, desires, goals, opinions, rights, preferences, and perspectives, and you do it because you fear rejection, conflict, or abandonment (Flett et al., 2007). Sometimes you may feel that you don't have a right to feel differently than your partner, your family, or your friends. Sometimes you may feel that it wouldn't make any difference to speak up. Sometimes you may feel you don't have a right to have a say in decisions, not even those that directly concern you. Sometimes you may feel you are too inept, uneducated, weak, or stupid for your perspective to be legitimate. You may have made such a habit of dismissing your own perspective that you are not even fully aware of yourself anymore, and are not completely aware that your voice has gone silent.

This inauthenticity in intimate relationships is usually marked by a strong belief that loving someone means that you always put your own needs last (Flett et al., 2007). Now, even women without a tendency toward depression will feel strongly that they should put their baby's needs first. This is not unusual, especially in the weeks and months after the birth of a baby (Thompson & Bendell, 2014), and it's hard to fault a new mother for feeling this way. However, over time, women who believe strongly that caring for others demands constant self-sacrifice find themselves depleted and unappreciated. We will discuss the benefits of caring for ourselves, and ways to do that, in future chapters. For now, however, it is important to note that feeling as if you are doing something wrong when you state your needs clearly and calmly, or that you are being selfish when you take time to take care of your own true needs, is a marker for the depression-prone woman (Flett et al, 2007).

Over time, women who do not express themselves genuinely in close relationships begin to feel as if their true self is markedly different from the person known by loved ones (Thompson & Bendell, 2014). These women end up feeling disconnected and angry. They may vacillate between just going along and erupting in angry hostility (Ussher, 2004).

Many women have never learned how to be real in their marriages or love relationships, their family relationships, or their friendships. What many women have seen modeled from other women their whole lives is that the highest values are to be nice, sweet, polite, and agreeable. If this describes you, you may not know what to do with your own opinions, your own anger, and your dissatisfaction with the status quo. If you do express any anger, you may explode into a rage after a prolonged time of suppressing it (Ussher, 2004). This may leave you feeling foolish and guilty. Such rages are seldom constructive or helpful, as they are at best ineffective, and at worst, do considerable damage.

Not everybody that self-silences is prone to the occasional volcanic eruption. This doesn't mean that there are no consequences to swallowing your real self whole. Self-silencing requires a really high level of vigilance over what you say, do, and express in body language. This constant self-monitoring is a constant drain on your personal resources, and can have serious consequences for both emotional and physical health (e.g., Nagurney, 2008).

Negative Attitudes Toward Motherhood

Depressed mothers as a group love their babies just as much as non-depressed mothers do, although they tend to have more negative attitudes about motherhood (Thompson & Bendell, 2014). Negative attitudes towards motherhood do not equal lack of love. Most of the negative attitudes toward motherhood that depression-prone women carry can be traced back to other depressive characteristics, some of which we have already discussed. If you are depression-prone, you may have rigidly high expectations of yourself as a mother, and you may feel that this is completely normal. It may not even occur to you that your expectations are unrealistically high.

Rigidly high expectations of yourself as a mother can lead to a sense of failure when the realities of new motherhood crash down upon you. Trying to do this new job of motherhood perfectly takes

Some expectations depression-prone moms may have of themselves are:

- *Good mothers want to always be with their children.*
- *Good mothers do not need to ask for help.*
- *Good mothers do not find motherhood difficult.*

If you, as a new mother, have set the bar so high, you may feel that you have failed the first test of motherhood if you ask for help (Thompson & Bendell, 2014).

the joy out of the experience. If the baby is fussy, or if there are medical problems to deal with, expecting yourself to do this job perfectly can lead to frustration or despair. It may lead to a feeling that life is restricted and difficult because of the baby. It may lead to unhappiness and even regret about deciding to have a baby (Thompson & Bendell, 2014).

Depression-prone women have usually had dissatisfying experiences in relationships already. You may believe that others expect you to be perfect. You may be in a relationship with critical or unsupportive people that confirm your negative beliefs about yourself. Even if your family is positive and supportive, you may be caught in negative patterns where you wear loved ones out seeking reassurance and affirmation repeatedly over the same issues. You may habitually silence your true self out of fear of rejection. You may create stress for yourself because your tools for coping with the challenges of life are inadequate. A history of these sorts of problems sets you up for negative expectations about the relationship with your baby. You can all too easily come to see the new baby as just another person that expects too much (Thompson & Bendell, 2014).

Repeating Patterns

Even when a relationship pattern is uncomfortable or painful, you will tend to repeat it until you recognize it and make conscious choices to change. Old relationship patterns are comfortable. You know what is expected of you. You know how to act. You know where you fit in the puzzle. You can predict what is going to happen and you feel like you have a measure of control.

You have a conscious mind and an unconscious mind. The conscious mind is whatever you are paying attention to at any given moment. It is good at precise problem-solving using a slow, stepwise, one-thing-at-a-time processor. The conscious mind communicates via thoughts and language (Collura, Zalaquett, Bonnstetter, & Chatters, 2014). The unconscious mind flows side by side with the conscious mind, a kind of background noise to whatever you are paying attention to. You become aware of the workings of your unconscious mind through bodily sensations connected to thoughts and impressions, or emotions. The unconscious mind is a quick-and-dirty parallel processor good at giving approximate answers practically instantaneously through an emotional reaction (Baumeister, Masicampo, & Vohs, 2011). This quick-and-dirty processing uses deeply encoded patterns based in your past experiences to come to its lightning-fast conclusions. Both the unconscious and the conscious parts of your mind have their uses (Collura, Zalaquett, Bonnstetter, & Chatters, 2014).

It is safe to say that you are barely aware of the myriad of decisions you have to make every day. If you had to get a precise answer to every one of them, directing your attention consciously to each tiny choice to make, your life would grind to a halt. You may know someone who has extreme difficulty making decisions: ordering from a menu, shopping for daily necessities, choosing a route to drive, or cleaning out the spare room all become agonizing processes. Everyone's life would be like this, and worse, if every small decision demanded a precise answer. The conscious mind is good at providing precise answers, but the time and attention required to give you those precise answers interrupts the flow of living (Collura et al., 2014).

There are times, however, when you really need to slow down and take the time to give this careful attention to decisions you are automatically making. Sometimes you can find yourself doing things and moving in directions that go against your own best interests. This is because emotional reactions based on the approximate answers provided by the unconscious mind are quicker than the deliberate reactions based on the slow and careful logic of the conscious mind. When it becomes apparent that the approximate answers of the unconscious mind are not good enough anymore, you need to consciously lay down new patterns.

You can upload your unconscious thoughts and impressions into your consciousness, so that you may examine and evaluate them (Baumeister et al., 2011). It tends to be a slow process that takes effort and skill. Often, people need support as they do this very important work. Without it, the quick-and-dirty unconscious processes will drive your emotions and influence you to repeat what is painfully familiar.

Conclusion

Over the course of your lifetime, the quality of your important relationships have been incorporated into your sense of self, as a community of voices. In turn, this sense of who you are has become a stable place within. You have a very human need to protect and confirm this stable place within. However, when your sense of self includes negativity and relentless self-criticism, protecting and confirming your stable place within leads to deeply depressing habits, such as relationship inauthenticity, toxic perfectionism, self-silencing, trying to merge your identity with someone else's, and viewing yourself as an object. These habitual ways of being operate on the automatic, unconscious level. They are not conscious choices that you make in the moment.

The good news is that humans are not only equipped with an automatic, unconscious mind, but also with a conscious, deliberate mind. Just because you aren't usually aware of the deep structures of your stable place within your own mind does not mean that you cannot become aware. This is good news! If you have become dissatisfied enough with the status quo, it is possible to shake it up. It is possible to insert more positive voices into the internal conversation, and to upset the balance of power so that negativity no longer reigns supreme.

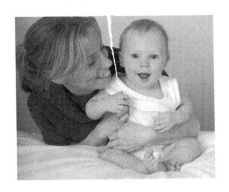

CHAPTER 5

The Keys to Change: Challenging Your Depression, Changing Your Patterns

One of my favorite movies of all times is Coal Miner's Daughter. *It is the story of country music legend, Loretta Lynn. In one scene, she has achieved incredible fame and success, and yet is struggling with anxiety, depression, and chronic headaches. Her breaking point comes when she can't remember the words to the songs in her show. She decides on an impulse to tell her audience just what she is going through. She said, "Patsy [Cline, Loretta's recently deceased best friend] used to say, 'little girl, you got to run your own life!' ... But my life's running me" (Apted & Schwartz, 1980). If you are struggling with depression, you know exactly what she was talking about.*

Your life has changed so much with the birth of your baby that contemplating more change may seem overwhelming. However, doing things the same old way is how you ended up depressed in the first place. So why not consider making some positive changes now that will benefit you and your child for years to come? Once you become convinced that you need some change, there is a systematic way to make it happen. These steps are endlessly repeatable, so you can carry them far into the future, continuing to tweak things about yourself and your life that are not working very well.

Key 1: Become Aware

If you only have a vague sense that you are not happy or that your life is not working for you, change will be a greater challenge. You must first sharpen your awareness of exactly what is not working. It is possible to habitually ignore your deepest wisdom. You can be in the midst of a full-blown depressive episode before it occurs to you that something is wrong.

You must first become aware of your own emotions. If you are in the habit of shutting your emotions down before they ever reach any level of conscious awareness, how can you examine them or learn to manage them better? It is possible to so deny painful feelings that they become anesthetized. Have you ever been insulted or otherwise treated unacceptably, and it was only later, when you thought about it, that you became irritated or angry? Have you ever had a loss, whether major or minor, in which you had a delayed sadness or grief reaction? These sorts of reactions are similar to when physical pain wakes up after anesthesia or painkilling medication begins to wear off. These are clues that you have developed the ability to anesthetize awareness of your emotions.

Most people are aware of the term "fight or flight response." Fight or flight refers to a natural system by which our system prepares to respond to danger. However, there are actually four possible responses to danger: fight, flight, freeze, and "tend or befriend" (e.g., Bracha, Ralston, Matsukawa, Williams, & Bracha, 2004; Taylor, 2006). A freeze response occurs in the immediate aftermath of severe stress, when you must evaluate the threat and orient yourself to the situation. Ever heard the phrase "deer in the headlights"? That refers to freezing. The numbing of natural emotional responses in stressful situations is also a kind of freeze response. It is sometimes called "being in shock," and when you are in crisis, it can be protective and keep you from becoming emotionally overloaded.

Feeling verbally or emotionally threatened by someone else can bring on a freeze response (Roelofs, Hagenaars, & Stins, 2010). The usefulness of the freeze response, however, is short-lived. It is important that you develop robust ways of coping with verbal or emotional threat, so that your sense of helplessness is reduced and you gain a sense of mastery over such situations. Since depression and a sense of helplessness go hand-in-hand, it is not hard to see why it is important to get beyond the freeze response.

"Tend and befriend" refers to a different sort of response to stress. It is more common in women than men, and can take the form of seeking approval from others, doing their bidding, accepting their perspectives, or stroking their egos, even, and maybe especially, when they are draining, domineering, critical, hurtful, or cruel (David & Lyons-Ruth, 2005).

If you are having a flashback to the discussion of the interpersonal behaviors of depression-prone people, you are on the right track. Excessive reassurance seeking, negative-feedback seeking, perfectionistic strivings, and self-silencing are complex human stress responses. Some symptoms of depression, such as fatigue, withdrawal, and low mood, may also be understood as an involuntary submissive response to chronic stress (Zuroff, Fournier, & Moskowitz, 2007). *Awareness* is the first key to reversing this pattern.

Psychotherapy

Psychotherapy, also called "talk therapy," is one way to increase awareness of your inner life. Quite aside from the expertise a therapist brings to the process, talking about your life, your relationships, and your inner experience brings a level of consciousness to living that just thinking can't compete with. Either individual or group psychotherapy can raise your level of awareness. The advantage of individual psychotherapy is that it is especially private, since the only people in the conversation are you and your therapist. The advantage of group psychotherapy is the support and insight you get from others going through something similar.

Mindfulness

Practicing *mindfulness* (Desrosiers, Vine, Klemanski, & Nolen-Hoeksema, 2013; Kang, Gruber, & Gray, 2013) promotes awareness as well. The opposite of *mindlessness,* mindfulness is the deliberate practice of being very present in each and every moment of life. There are many ways to bring a mindful awareness into your daily experience. Setting aside some time each day for mindfulness meditation is one way. Mindfulness meditation consists of quieting the body and taking charge of your capacity to pay attention. The attention is turned inward to noticing, in exquisite detail, the experience of being here, at this moment and in this space, in your body, and as yourself. The sensations of the breath, of pain or of comfort, of temperature, pressure, movement, sound, light, and smell are noticed and attended to without judgment.

To meditate mindfully without judgment means to let go of self-criticism and making value judgments about your experience. Sometimes, mindfulness meditation may consist of turning the attention to an object, such as a piece of chocolate, a raisin, a beautiful flower, or a blade of grass. You may find it helpful to use a recording or podcast, in which you follow a guided mindfulness meditation.

Another way to practice mindfulness is to choose at least one activity per day to engage in mindfully. This may be eating, bathing or showering, breastfeeding, taking a walk, or any of the many activities you do every day in a mindless manner. Give any or all of the mundane activities of life your undivided attention. Just for the time it takes to take your bath, eat your lunch, breastfeed your baby, walk your dog, or sew on a button, rest from planning the future or fretting about the past. For that moment, be one with what you are doing. Experience the moment. Be mindful in it.

Body Scanning

Mentally scanning your body at regular intervals also helps develop self-awareness. Starting at the top of your head and moving slowly and deliberately down to your toes, just notice how each part of your body feels.

As you get into a habit of mentally scanning your body when you are in a calm state, it will become more natural to do this when something stressful or upsetting is happening. This exercise can be especially helpful in recognizing how you feel when you are with different people. How do you feel after you have spent an hour with your sister, mother, or in-laws? How do you feel during an afternoon with your husband? How do you feel when left alone with your baby?

As you gain practice in self-awareness, you will begin to notice thoughts and emotions bubbling to the surface. Notice them, but do not critique them. Judging them to be "good" or "bad," as feelings you "should" or "should not" have, as "reasonable" or "unreasonable," is counterproductive. What is important in this first step is simply awareness itself. Tell yourself, "I just had this thought," or "I feel this way," but resist putting a value judgment on it. If you are in the habit of criticizing or evaluating every thought and feeling, not doing that will be a challenge. Start with a simple willingness to observe without forming an opinion. Become aware of the constant evaluation that you impose, even upon your thoughts and feelings. Practice awareness that passing judgment on yourself is something to recognize and then release. Let it go (Kang, Gruber & Gray, 2013).

You may find it helpful to have a bodily gesture for releasing self-criticism when you recognize you are doing it. This could involve taking a deep breath and blowing it out through your mouth, in your imagination blowing away your self-criticism. You might make a wiping motion with your hands. Although there is nothing powerful or magical about the gesture itself, when done mindfully it can help you release self-criticism and let it go.

Journaling

Another way to become aware of your inner life is to journal. A password-protected word processing file on your computer will work. If you are a good typist, then you may be able to write almost as fast as you can think. Do not censor yourself. Instead, write about what you are thinking and feeling in the moment. Reread it. Add to it and modify it if you wish. If the thoughts and feelings that bubble to the surface are about particular relationships, you can turn a journal entry into a letter to a loved one. The letter does not need to be sent; it just needs to express what you would like to say. Say what you would say if you could be completely honest and there would be no repercussions.

Dreaming

Still another way to become more aware of your inner life is to take your dreams seriously. Keep a notebook or pad of paper and a pen beside your bed. A tablet computer would work too. Write down your dreams as soon as you wake up. Muse on the major themes that crop up. The more you pay attention to your dreams, the more likely you are to remember them. You dream every night, although you may not usually remember it. Some dreams reflect the process of going over the events of the day and consolidating them into memory. Others are more enigmatic, containing symbolism and emotional material that takes time and thought to unravel. Still others feel prophetic and otherworldly. All are part of you and deserve your attention during the waking hours.

Face Your Fears

There may be a certain amount of fear that comes with facing what is going on beneath the surface. You may fear that in recognizing your anger, it will rage out of control. You may fear that in recognizing your grief and devastation, it will consume you. It is important to remember that thoughts and emotions have no power outside of the power you choose to give them. In becoming aware, you take the first step towards managing them. I do not say control them, because that would imply that you can just make them go away or forcibly change them. Managing them, on the other hand, implies making reasonable decisions about what you will do with the information they supply.

Key 2: Challenge The Status Quo

Thoughts, feelings, and behaviors are intimately related to one another. They form a system in which each element exerts an influence over the other elements. Each contributes to the downward spiral of depression, and each has a role in recovery.

Change always involves risk. You are very good at what you are doing now. After all, you have been doing it for years. Whether it is being so agreeable that eventually you explode in rage, or stuffing your grief and pain until it makes you sick, or putting up a wall of overwork or prickliness to keep others at bay, you are good at it. You know how it works and you know what you can expect. On the other hand, if you haven't tried calm but clear communication with your partner, saying no to unreasonable demands from your family, or protecting yourself from those that hurt you, you do not know if you can do it. You are almost sure not to be good at it when you first start trying. It won't be automatic and you will have to give it your thought and attention.

Challenge yourself to consider:
- *What would happen if you changed the way you think?*
- *What would happen if you changed the way you behave?*
- *What would happen if your feelings changed?*
- *Could you tolerate the changes?*
- *What would you have to give up?*
- *What would you gain?*

What if you could change your baby's life for the better by handling your depression? If you haven't been willing to change the status quo for yourself, are you are willing to do it for your baby? Relieving your current depression, and reducing your chances of having another episode, can have a profound impact on your relationship with your baby, her development, and the quality of your family life for many years to come (Nylen, Moran, Franklin, & O'Hara, 2006).

When you fly in an airplane, the flight attendant gives you instructions on what to do in case there is a loss of cabin pressure. If oxygen masks drop down from the ceiling, passengers travelling with children are instructed to first put the mask over their own faces and then to secure the oxygen mask for their child. This is because the time needed to put on your own mask is minimal and not likely to have any bad results for your child. However, if you pass out because you haven't taken care of yourself, who is going to care for your child? An additional thought is that putting on an oxygen mask may be scary for a child. If their parent is wearing one, the scariness is reduced because the parent is modeling that it is safe. This is a metaphor for caring for yourself. You must care for yourself, not because you are selfish, but because you have responsibilities. Caring for yourself is a way of caring for your child. When you care for yourself, you model that self-care is important. In caring for yourself, you will teach yourself healthier patterns of thoughts, feelings, and of interacting in relationships, and you will pass that on to the next generation through example.

Perhaps you have very good reasons for not challenging the status quo. The only question left to ask is, are there even better reasons to change?

Key 3: Experiment with Something New

Now we get down to the specifics of your situation. What is it that is not working for you? Does it have to do with your marriage relationship? Family relationships? Friendships? Is it your relationship with yourself? Whatever it is, get very clear in your own mind what part of the problem belongs to you and what belongs to someone else.

Imagine yourself standing in the center of a big circle drawn on the floor. This circle is just big enough that you can fully extend your arms at shoulder height and your fingertips will be directly above it. This is the zone that belongs to you. When you move, this circle moves with you. Now imagine the circle extending upwards, forming a clear dome that encloses you from head to foot. The dome marks the boundary between yourself and other people. It is similar to a cell wall. A cell wall marks what the cell is and what it is not, but it is permeable. It very selectively allows things in and out, such as nutrients and waste products.

Plug the Leaks in Your Boundaries

Depression-prone people tend to have leaky interpersonal boundaries. Leaky boundaries happen when you are unsure about what is your responsibility and what is not, when you give too much of your own power away, and there is too much energy going out. Your boundaries are also leaky when you allow others to inhabit your personal zone and intrude upon you (Jacobvitz, Hazen, Curran, & Hitchens, 2004).

Getting very clear, inside yourself, about what is and is not *you* helps you to plug up the leaks in your boundaries. Remember that the only person you can control is yourself. However, you *can* control yourself. That's it. You can't make other people *do* or *feel* or *think* anything. This includes your baby. It is an invaluable lesson to learn right now, when your baby is so tiny, that you cannot *make* her do anything. She is her own person. You can help her develop desirable behavior and impose reasonable consequences for misbehavior, but that is still what *you* do. She gets to decide whether she wants to be cooperative or to take the consequences.

If this is true for your baby, who for many years will desperately need you for her very survival, then it is many more times true for others. Release them to find their own paths. Those paths may intertwine with yours, and it is a joy when two or more people choose to cooperate with one another and to accommodate one another's needs. However, each person

- *Depression-prone people often have trouble telling other people no, giving in too much for too long, and eventually being harsh and explosive in reaction to feeling violated or disrespected.*

- *Depression-prone people tend to feel responsible for other people's feelings, and to place responsibility for their own feelings on others. This confusion explains why depression-prone people may waffle between being overly agreeable and being hostile. This hostility can be open and obvious, such as outbursts of rage or vindictiveness, but most often involves using stealth and manipulation.*

retains the right and responsibility to make his or her own choices. It can be very freeing to realize that you are not ultimately responsible for the choices others make.

Relinquish Control Over Others

Ask yourself if you have been trying to control anyone else through aggressive or manipulative tactics. Aggression is a direct use of force, such as physical violence, screaming and cursing, or destruction of property. It is important for you to get any tendency you have towards aggression under control. Seek out help and support for your own aggression, and keep your distance from others who are aggressive with you. Whether it is you or someone you love that is engaging in aggressive tactics, everyone involved must become physically safe before emotional progress can be made. Do whatever you must do to get yourself and your baby to safety. Have a plan in place to insure everyone's safety if you yourself are struggling with aggressive behaviors.

Manipulation, by contrast, is using underhanded or sneaky methods to coerce people into doing something they would not otherwise do (e.g., Grieve, 2011). Manipulative tactics include saying things to induce guilt in other people, twisting the facts to get an emotional reaction or to get others to change their minds, self-pity, withholding love or affection, and giving others the silent treatment. You may recognize manipulative behaviors easily when they are described if you have often been on the receiving end. It may be harder, though, to recognize when they are happening to you in the moment. It is well worth the effort to recognize when others are attempting to manipulate you, and to be very aware that how you respond to this manipulation is your choice. Is this really behavior that you want to reward? Rewarding bad behavior only makes it stronger.

It can be extremely challenging to recognize when you yourself are manipulating others, but remember that manipulation is ultimately destructive. Manipulation is hurtful, and wastes your energy trying to control other people, who are not your property to control. Instead, concentrate on yourself, your own behaviors, and your own feelings.

Give Up Mind-Reading

Families and relationships that spend lots of time and energy trying to control one another are usually characterized by a basic but unspoken assumption; that people can read each other's minds. Remember the discussion of anxious attachment, and how someone who has formed an anxious attachment tries to predict and control the other person. People focused on controlling one another are constantly involved in a mutual dance in which everyone believes that they can know what everyone else feels and thinks (Asen & Fonagy, 2012).

Of course sometimes we know from experience what our partner, or a family member, **probably** thinks about a given subject or how they are *likely* to react. This is part of what it means to be close. However, when this mindreading assumption becomes overblown, closeness turns into control and smothering. It can result in total relationship ruptures. People are complex, and we can't know everything about anyone. People also change and grow. When we keep

*If you feel as if your life has spun out of control, or that your partner or someone else wants to control you, then it is crucial to first get very clear in your mind that **you** are in control of your **own** decisions and your **own** actions. Focus your energies on the choices you do have, and let go of the rest. Imagine yourself inside a clear protective dome, responsible only for your own actions. Imagine others in the same way. Release your loved ones in your mind. You are only responsible for yourself.*

ourselves from acting on assumptions that may or may not be true, we give others the space to be themselves and to make different choices. The relationship itself may change and grow.

Experiment with new ways of being with other people based on the assumptions that people cannot read one another's minds and that each individual human being is responsible only for himself or herself. Try saying, "Let me think about it" when it feels as if someone is trying to force you into an immediate decision. Tell them that if you must give them an immediate answer, then you will for sure say "no" to whatever they want. If, after someone has been to see the baby or spoken to you on the phone, you realize that you are hurt by something they did or said, try informing them calmly that you found their words or actions hurtful. State that you believe you deserve to be treated respectfully. If you have been practicing this by writing in your journal, such as writing letters to those who have frequently hurt you, telling the actual person will be easier.

Set Limits with Others

It is empowering to realize that you have every right to set limits with others. Although you may be feeling angry, anger is not required for you to set limits. Because intense anger flows from a sense of hurt and powerlessness, the power that comes from asserting your right to set limits will tend to reduce your anger's intensity.

Demonstrate respectfulness in your words and tone, not groveling or submission. If you are confident that you have done this to the best of your ability, recognize that the other person's reaction is his or her choice. Some people will be apologetic and horrified that they hurt you. Others will be hostile and angry. Still others will withdraw.

You may be able to predict the other person's reaction with a fair degree of accuracy, but you will never know with complete certainty until you take action. If you expect the other person to go on the attack, be prepared with some words of affirmation for yourself:

- I am a human being worthy of respect and nurture.

- I must learn to stand up for myself so that I can be a role model for my baby.

- I stand up for myself in defiance of my depression.

In a sense, telling the other person directly that they have hurt you is only fair. It is giving them a chance to acknowledge it and make amends. If they choose hostility or withdrawal instead, that is their choice. At least you will know for sure.

Reexamine Your Roles

Do you have roles or responsibilities in your family, your job, or your life that are not working for you? Perhaps you have taken on these because once you enjoyed them, because you thought that other people expected you to do them, or because you thought no one else could do them correctly.

A new baby is a great reason to reexamine how you spend your time and energy, and to reorder your life according to your deepest and most enduring values. This will require exercising your limit-setting skills, with yourself and with others. Healthy boundaries permit us to make positive choices about what to let into our personal space and what to keep out. It is a highly individualized process, which is a reason why personal awareness has been emphasized so much up to this point. It is also a highly flexible process, because your needs and values will change over time. When you say "yes" to something, you say "no" to something else. When you do choose to say "yes," be very intentional in your choice.

Summary

Just as a cell wall has certain rules for what goes out and what comes in, your interpersonal boundaries set up rules for what you will do and what you will tolerate. Depression symptoms are a sign that there is a problem with these rules. You may have been spending too much of your energy trying to control others, and not enough time setting limits with others who want to control you. Too much energy has been going out and too many toxins have been allowed in. You may have been saying "yes" to the wrong things and "no" to the right things. Changing the rules with yourself and others takes time, effort, and a willingness to have others be unhappy with you.

Key 4: Evaluate

Constructing and maintaining an appropriate boundary system involves a lot of skill. If you already had these skills, you probably would have been using them all along. When you first start telling people "no" and setting limits with them, concentrating on controlling yourself rather than other people, and when you start living your life based on your most authentic goals and values, you are bound to face some obstacles along the way.

You may find that there are some people who pay no attention to your first attempts at telling them "no." Your mother comes over anyway, after being told it's not a good time. Your husband continues to criticize, despite being told you find it hurtful. A coworker gives you unsolicited advice about being the perfect mother, despite being told that you would rather find your own mothering style. These do not represent failure on your part. They represent growth. All of these situations are opportunities to learn more about effective boundary setting. In some cases, the "no" simply has to be repeated often enough that it finally gets through. This is most often the case with people who truly care and want the best for you, but are not accustomed to you taking control of your own life. They have gotten in the habit of steamrolling over you, and it may take a while for them to get the message.

In other cases, you may need to impose consequences for those that ignore your personal boundaries. This is for those who are not getting the message, especially those who are malicious or who fill your life with drama. Consequences may involve screening your calls, texts, and doorbell, literally walking away from the conversation, or keeping any contact brief and to the point. Consequences are always about what you *will* or *won't* do, and involve "if-then" propositions. "If he does X, then I will do Y." You do not have to announce this to the other person. You just have to tell it to yourself. Announcing the consequences for bad behavior will just antagonize some people.

Getting good at setting personal boundaries is, to a certain extent, a trial-and-error proposition. First, you clarify to yourself what you will and won't tolerate from others. You identify what is your responsibility and what is the other person's. Then you communicate your boundaries clearly to the person who is violating them, and observe what happens. Lastly, you evaluate the effectiveness of stating your boundaries. If just taking a stand is ineffective, you impose some consequences for continued boundary violations.

You must actually and consistently follow through with the consequences, otherwise your boundaries simply become idle threats. Idle threats are not boundaries. Idle threats are annoyances that strong-willed people crash through. Sometimes, you will fail in your resolve to impose needed consequences on boundary violators. This is part of the learning process. You will pick up the phone when you had resolved let it go to voicemail. You will cry and argue rather than walking away from mean-spirited criticism. Don't give up! Instead, step back and evaluate what you did and did not do. Decide what you are going to do the next time.

> *Self-criticism says, "I should have known better."*
>
> *Evaluation says, "I can learn from this."*

The step of evaluation turns what once may have left you feeling defeated into a learning opportunity. Evaluation is not the same thing as self-criticism. Self-criticism operates from the principle of "I should have known better." Evaluation operates from the principle of "I can learn from this." So sometimes your attempts at setting and maintaining boundaries don't turn out so well. Expect this. It is all part of the process.

Key 5: Recruit Support

You may struggle with maintaining confidence in your own perspective, especially with close family members or with people who are pushy or controlling. Because people fit like locks-and-keys in close relationships, if you experience a lot of self-doubt, you are likely to be in relationship with at least some people who have an overabundance of ego. You may be in relationship with people who have problems seeing anyone's perspective but their own. It can be very helpful to recruit support from a third party to help you maintain your perspective with these individuals.

Let's say you find your sister to be bossy and controlling, and you are dreading her visit to see the baby because you expect her to burden you with unsolicited advice and expect you to follow her orders. At the same time, there are good things about her and you are not ready to totally cut her out of your life. In situations like this, recruiting an ally to be present can be very helpful. Choose someone that you feel confident has your best interests at heart. Hopefully, this is your partner, although this is not the case for everyone.

Often, difficult people are on their best behavior when there is a third person present. At the very least, the presence of a supportive third person gives you a witness that will help bolster your confidence in your own perspective. Recruiting a willing ally can also be helpful when others are attempting to pressure you into an immediate decision, even if your ally is not actually present at the time. It is important not to abdicate your personal power to anyone, including a well-meaning supporter. However, if you can truly say, "That's something I need to discuss with my partner first," or, "I'll need to ask the pediatrician about that first," by all means, say it. Major life decisions that would affect partners must, after all, be discussed with them. Decisions on practices that could affect your baby's health or well-being are truly best made after consultation with her doctor. Whether you actually discuss it with them, or go about your business without bothering with the issue further, is up to you.

It is important to distinguish recruiting support from asking someone else to fight your battles for you, or asking them to rescue you from difficult situations. Having a supportive third party present is only helpful to the extent that they help you stay grounded in your own perspective and provide a witness to what transpires. It is still up to you to define and enforce the boundaries with difficult people.

97

Sometimes, the people with whom it is the most challenging to establish good boundaries are those that engage in stealth tactics. Stealth tactics are things like:

- *inflicting verbal jabs while denying any hurtful intentions,*

- *accusing you of being overly sensitive,*

- *engaging in circular logic, or*

- *saying you are crazy or hormonal when you challenge them.*

Sometimes, particularly difficult people will spread highly skewed versions of your conversation, to the point of inventing things or attributing something they said to you. Such tactics can be crazy-making, and having a supportive witness present can help tremendously.

Psychotherapy is another way to recruit support for the changes you desire to make. In addition to the benefits mentioned before, such as being a time and space for you to become more aware of your thoughts and feelings, psychotherapy is a consistent source of support for making positive changes in your life. In psychotherapy, you can discuss your relationship patterns almost in real time.

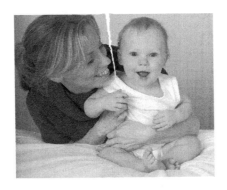

CHAPTER 6

Creating an Anchor Within: Practices to Combat Depression

I have named depression "the pit." When you are in that dark place, it does feel as if you are in a deep, dark hole. Understanding how you got depressed in the first place is like getting your bearings, and learning which way is up. However, that is only part of the solution. What you need next are materials and tools to build a ladder out. The basics to building that ladder have been discussed in the last chapter: awareness, challenging the status quo, experimenting with something new, evaluating your progress, and recruiting support. Some practical ways to bring those basics into your life have already been discussed. This chapter will give you more tools for your ladder into recovery.

Some of the tools discussed here are "body-primary" and others are "mind-primary" practices. You can't really divide the body and mind into two units that are treated separately, but one or the other is usually the primary target in any given method. Be sure you are dividing your efforts to heal between body-primary and mind-primary tools. Try something in each category. Body-primary tools focus on healing from the physiological effects of depression. Mind-primary modalities focus on healing from the mental and emotional damage.

Body-Primary Practices

Slumber Care

A newborn in the house disrupts everybody's sleep, and during the third trimester of pregnancy you may not have been sleeping so well either. Unfortunately, depression adds to many women's difficulty sleeping. You may be too tense and restless to sleep when the baby does, or you may not be able to return to sleep after a nighttime feeding. You may wake up spontaneously in the wee hours of the morning, after a few hours of disturbed sleep, full of anxiety dreams.

Nursing and Sleeping Arrangements

Depressed or not, you are more likely to have an emotional meltdown when you are sleep deprived. Figuring out ways to increase the quantity and quality of your sleep is vital to returning to an emotional even keel. Contrary to what others may tell you, there is increasing evidence that exclusively breastfeeding mothers get more sleep, get better sleep, and feel more refreshed and alert during the day (Kendall-Tackett, Cong & Hale, 2011). So if you are breastfeeding, don't quit! Also, keep the baby close to you at night. Keeping her in a bassinet or cradle within arm's reach means that you don't have to actually get out of bed to nurse her in the middle of the night. Being able to check on her by putting your hand on her in the dark is apt to reduce your anxiety. It may even help reduce her risk of SIDS (McKenna & McDade, 2005).

When our second son was born, my husband and I finally got our nighttime baby care routine down to a fine art. We kept a brown paper bag at the end of our bed, and the top rolled down so that it held itself open and upright. I kept the baby in his cradle on my side of the bed, and my husband had a supply of diapers and wipes on his side. When the baby awakened for a feeding, I scooped him up and passed him to his dad, who changed his diaper and re-dressed him. He then passed the baby back to me, and would toss the rolled-up wet diaper long-distance into the paper bag in the dark. This maximized our sleep and minimized the disruption. Avoiding turning on the lights or noisemakers like the television also sent the baby the message that it was nighttime, which helped him adapt his wake-sleep rhythms more quickly.

Release Toxic Perfectionism

Sleep and rest is a major area impacted by perfectionism and poor communication with others. If you think other people expect perfection from you, it will be harder to ask for help and harder to receive it. You will tend to feel guilty for not being Supermom. It will be harder to relax, rest, and sleep. This actually prolongs your exhaustion and the time it takes to recover. Remind yourself that everyone needs help and that help is good—with the possible exception of help that comes with strings attached. Help is better when it comes freely and without obligation to the other person or an expectation that they can now violate your personal boundaries. You will need the good kind of help so you can catch up on your sleep and avoid the sleep-deprivation meltdowns. In the first few weeks, napping is fine to help you recover from labor and delivery. As time goes on, however, limiting your sleep during the day can help to reset your inner clock and help you get better quality sleep at night.

Also, try some of the relaxation methods described in this chapter. Try them before bed or when you wake up in the middle of the night.

Stress-Busting

Anxiety is a combination of worrying, muscle tension, and physiological arousal that leads to a variety of other problems, including insomnia, avoiding important life activities, and physical symptoms (American Psychiatric Association, 2013). Anxiety and depression go hand-in-hand, and when you're depressed, a systematic way of encouraging your body and mind to relax can go a long way to making you feel better. Since, at first, worry can seem uncontrollable, and relaxing your mind can seem like an impossible task, relaxing the body can be the most practical way to start.

Progressive Relaxation

Progressive relaxation forces physical relaxation by systematically tiring out your voluntary muscles. At first, choose the quietest spot you have available. Your desk at work or a short break in a restroom stall will do in a pinch. If possible, put on some gentle music, nature sounds, or white noise. Use earbuds if necessary. Take a moment to allow your body to calm down from any upsetting or stressful moments.

Tense each muscle group in your body for a few seconds at a time, until they are tired. Start with tensing to a slow count of 5 to 10, increasing the time as needed. Then release and feel your muscles relax. A tired muscle can't hold tension so well. Begin with the muscles of your face. Move, next, to the muscles of the neck and shoulders, and then to the arms, down to the fingertips. Then work on your abdominals. Continue until each part of the body has been intensely contracted and released. Notice how you felt before and how you feel afterward. Notice how long it takes for each muscle group to begin to tire. Notice how intensely you must contract each muscle group to get a relaxation response. Remember to breathe slowly and deeply throughout the exercise. Wiggle a little in your seat afterwards to make sure everything is good and loose.

Once you get the hang of it, this exercise can be done anywhere-- driving in the car, or even while feeding or diapering your baby. Well, as long as you skip the part where you squeeze your eyes closed! Any time you feel your body carrying tension, a few minutes devoted to progressive relaxation can help you feel a lot better.

Deep Breathing

It sounds simple, but it actually takes some practice. Everybody breathes, but when you are tense and anxious, your breath becomes shallow and rapid. Deep breathing is deliberately concentrating on your breath, becoming aware of how it changes when you become anxious or upset, and purposefully making it slower and deeper. The slower part is crucial, because you don't want to hyperventilate. Hyperventilation can make you feel lightheaded and dizzy, which generally doesn't help you relax. For the span of 5 to 10 breaths, don't think about anything but breathing. If you find your thoughts wandering, do not berate yourself, just redirect them calmly back to your breath.

Massage

Therapeutic touch is good for babies, and it's good for moms too. It has been demonstrated to alleviate depression symptoms as well as anxiety, and even ADHD. The benefits of an hour-long massage can last all week (Field, Diego, & Hernandez-Reif, 2007). Find a massage therapist that is reputable and that you trust, so that you can completely relax while on the table.

If you can't afford a professional massage, buy a book or read up on massage techniques on the internet, and practice what you learn on your partner. Be sure your partner learns and practices on you, too! In a pinch, a shiatsu pillow can help work out some kinks. However, the clearest benefits come with professional massage, so that your whole body gets a safe and thorough workout.

Sensory Experiences

Approach relaxation from the sensory angle. Make a list of sensory experiences that you find relaxing. I designed my therapy office to maximize relaxation, with a soothing color on the walls, soothing art, a scented wax warmer, soft lighting, and white noise to filter outside noises. I try to use every sensory modality to induce relaxation. You can do this too, in your home or office.

Scents

What smells or scents put you into a relaxed and happy mood? If you are not sure, take a stroll into a candle store or one that sells scented lotions and creams. A friend told me that when she gets anxious, she goes into her laundry room and sniffs the good-smelling laundry soap! Peppermint hand cream has become a signature item in my therapy office. The majority of women who come through my door find it comforting. I also find the smell of fresh wood to be soothing, especially cedar. It reminds me of Christmas trees and my grand-mother's cedar wardrobe.

Water

Water, in all of its forms, can be used to induce relaxation. A warm bath, complete with soft music and candles, can be just the ticket for insomnia. A hot shower, with the spray focused on tense shoulders, can help your whole body unwind. One of my favorite relaxation experiences is floating in a quiet backyard pool on a raft under the stars. A tabletop fountain with its soft bubbling sound, a tall glass of ice water, or just the sound of flowing water using a nature sounds app on your smartphone can help you de-stress.

Sunlight

While overexposure to the sun can cause sunburn, do not discount the benefits of moderate exposure to natural light. Some women's depression is worse during the dark months of the year, and improves during the spring and summer (American Psychiatric Association, 2013). Try a regular brisk walk around the block during daylight hours, working in your yard, or just sitting by an open sunny window for a few minutes a day.

Textures

Texture is another way to incorporate positive sensory experiences into your daily life. A friend of mine says she likes to touch the cool, slick surface of her granite countertops when she is feeling tense. It calms her right down. Popping bubble wrap, fingering a worry stone in your pocket, or wrapping yourself in a favorite quilt are all ways of using texture to de-stress. Have a few go-to methods for soothing yourself when things get rough.

Working It Out

Yoga

Yoga is a terrific mind-body discipline that combines the benefits of meditation and exercise. It has also been shown to help reduce the symptoms of depression in perinatal women. For those that find themselves at first too jittery and distracted to meditate, yoga engages your body and gives you something very concrete to do as you learn to still your mind. If you are just beginning to try yoga, it may be best to go to a class led by a qualified instructor. There are options for self-guided yoga, such as yoga DVDs or online courses, but you don't get personal feedback from these. The social contact that comes with a class may be beneficial to you, too.

Exercise

Exercise can not only help you lose the baby weight and regain muscle tone, but it can brighten your mood. The key is getting started. If you choose to walk, just tell yourself that all you are obligated to do is to put on your shoes and walk for five minutes. If you choose to exercise following a DVD, all you are obligated to do is get out your mat, pop in the disc, and participate for five minutes. If you feel like continuing, then do. If you want to quit, you are permitted to quit. Of course, quitting won't help you feel better or get you into shape, but chances are, once you get started you will want to finish your workout.

When you are depressed, getting started is the biggest obstacle to exercise. It's worth the effort though, because over time, exercise has been shown to be as effective as antidepressant medication in relieving a depressed mood (Daley, 2008).

Medication

Antidepressants may not be the total answer, but they can be part of the answer. The life changes discussed in this book are not a quick fix, but are rather part of a process that may take a while. Antidepressant medications, on the other hand, can help you feel better much more quickly. The combination of antidepressants and psychotherapy for depression is a particularly potent combination. The rule of thumb is this: meds work faster, therapy works longer (Cuijpers et al., 2014).

Often, part of being depressed is feeling as if you have brain fog, with poor concentration, low energy, and very little motivation. It is very hard to gain insight into your inner life when you are foggy and tired all the time. The addition of an appropriate antidepressant medication to your regimen can help you gain the mental clarity to work on your thoughts and your relationships.

Have a talk with your physician if you decide you would like a trial of antidepressant medication. Not all antidepressants are safe to take while you are nursing, but most are (see www.InfantRisk. org). Also, it is important to take your medications as prescribed and to consult your physician if you decide to discontinue them. An antidepressant is not necessarily something you will have to stay on for the rest of your life, but should not be stopped and started whimsically without medical guidance.

Regard any antidepressant medication prescribed for you as part of your recovery, not the whole answer. If you are going to psychotherapy, try to find a therapist who is willing to work closely with your physician. In some settings, such as programs for postpartum depression based in teaching hospitals or clinics, you may have the benefit of an entire treatment team to help coordinate the various aspects of your care. In other settings, however, you may have to put the various professionals in touch with one another yourself.

Diet and Dietary Supplements

There are a million different opinions out there on healthy ways to eat. This can be a real problem for a new mother who is perfection-istic, a characteristic that may propel you towards trying to find and adhere to the "perfect eating system" or "perfect diet." The result may either be rigidity that becomes overwhelming and stressful, or totally giving up and diving into the nearest bag of potato chips. As in other aspects of life, releasing toxic perfectionism when it comes to what you eat can be an important part of emotional healing.

Because depression is not only a psychological condition expressed in emotional and behavioral symptoms, but also a medical condition expressed by underlying physical inflammation, lifestyle choices can impact your recovery. As in other aspects of your recovery, however, gradual and thoughtful change is preferable to radical change that usually will prove unsustainable.

Professional Nutrition Advice

If you are willing to seek the help of a physician or a psychotherapist, why not add at least one session with a nutritionist or registered dietitian? You can get personalized advice on meeting your nutri-tional goals, such as recovering from depression, losing excess baby weight, or regaining your pre-pregnancy level of fitness.

In the meantime, changing your nutritional habits with the goal of helping your depression should focus on what you can add rather than what you take away. Good first steps might be adding a multivitamin and increasing your water intake. Concentrate on maximizing your intake of nutrients within an acceptable calorie limit. Get the most nutritional bang for your calorie buck. Even if you have other medical conditions that demand dietary restrictions, this goal to maximize your nutrition should be achievable.

Mindful Eating

Mindful eating is an important way to improve your diet while you are working on your depression. Remember that mindfulness is the opposite of mindlessness. Mindful eating means that you engage in a thoughtful practice of paying attention to every aspect of what, how, when, where, and why you are eating. Have regular meals and planned snacks, and sit at the table using a real plate and real silverware. Preferably, eat the meal with your partner and any older children you have. Notice how your food looks, how hot it is, how it tastes, how it smells, and how it feels in your mouth. Slow down, chew it well, and pause between bites. Avoid allowing yourself to get so ravenously hungry between meals that you have trouble eating mindfully. My grandfather, who was always rail-thin and who remained strong and active into his 90s, made a personal habit of eating an apple before every meal so that he would not be tempted to overeat. I am amazed at his lifelong wisdom and restraint.

Setting rigid goals, such as losing the baby weight within a short time frame or adhering to a radically different diet, are likely to increase your stress and be counterproductive. Try some small changes. Make them even smaller, if necessary. If you can't manage eating three meals a day, plus two snacks mindfully, what about being mindful for one meal a day, or for one snack? Small steps in the right direction will eventually add up.

Fish Oil

While you are consulting with your dietitian, or with your physician about medication, also discuss the benefits of dietary supplements: what you should be trying, how much and how often to take it. Evidence is accumulating that omega-3 fatty acids, eicosapentaenoic acid (EPA) and docosahexaenoic acid (DHA), nutrients contained in the oils of cold-water fish, are helpful in reducing inflammation associated with perinatal depression. Fish oil supplements containing these nutrients are generally considered safe for use while you are breastfeeding (Kendall-Tackett, 2010).

The U.S. Pharmacoepia (www.USP.org), a non-industry-based organization, independently rates the safety of fish oil products. Check out their website for the listing of products they verify. The dosage for depression is 1,000 mg EPA and 200 to 400 mg of DHA.

Mind-Primary Practices

Mindfulness Meditation

Learning to practice mindfulness has been shown to decrease symptoms of depression and anxiety in perinatal women. Mothers that have learned to practice mindfulness also have seen improvements in their relationships with their children (Snyder, Shapiro, & Treleaven, 2012). The basics of mindfulness meditation have already been explained in the previous chapter. At its essence, mindfulness is about living in the present moment, rather than living the future in anxiety or the past in depression (Snyder et al., 2012). It is about cultivating awareness of both your inner and outer life. Setting aside time each day for mindfulness meditation is an important way to do that. Mindfulness meditation helps to clear your mind and bring yourself mentally and physically into the present time and space.

If you ever just feel like running away from home, mindfulness meditation actually is a healthy way to do that. The time spent in mindfulness meditation is time that you release your tight grip on all the burdens of life, and take charge of your attention (Snyder et al., 2012).

During some meditative times, you may focus on your breath, or on the state and workings of your own body. Focus on attending to internal sensations, such as the beating of your heart, or sensations such as heat, cold, pressure, air movement, and texture against your skin. Take this time to train your attention to live moment by moment in your body. This may be a challenge if you are accustomed to living in your head (Snyder et al., 2012).

During other meditative times, you may focus on an external object, such as a piece of artwork, a flower, or a piece of fruit. These times help you to focus on something other than your internal sensations. Skillfully tacking between attention to the internal and attention to the external is an important part of managing your emotions well (Snyder et al., 2012).

Mindfulness is not just for the time of day set aside for meditation. Your meditative time is intended to leak over into the rest of your day. It is about being very present mentally and emotionally in every bodily act. So take your developing powers of observation, of both internal and external stimuli, into every activity. Mindfulness shrinks the worry and stewing over many things that characterize both anxiety and depression, and expands your present moment. (Snyder et al., 2012).

Prayer

Similar but not identical to meditative practice, prayer is your very individual practice of connecting to God (or whatever your name for the Eternal, the Infinite, the Almighty). Even if you believe strongly in prayer, your actual prayer practice may have shut down as you have become more and more depressed. You may be avoiding introspection and reflection. It is time to deliberately open up those streams again, in the interest of reducing your symptoms of depression (Denny, 2011). Choose a beautiful prayer used often in your faith tradition. Read it and speak it aloud often. Think about its meaning. Add your own spontaneous prayers to it. Find versions of it set to music.

Prayer may not be something everyone adds to their daily lives. However, if it holds meaning and importance to you, don't allow any tendency to avoid introspection to rob you of it. It is a conundrum that depression brings overwhelming self-criticism, a destructive form of introspection, and yet, often depressed people avoid introspection's more helpful forms.

Journaling

Journaling was mentioned in the previous chapter, but it important enough and powerful enough to talk about in even more depth. It is an effective way to combat depression, probably because it provides a way to develop awareness of your inner life (Stice, Burton, Bearman, & Rohde, 2007). There are no rules to journaling, except to do it. You may wish to journal only when you are very emotionally upset and need to express yourself in a safe manner. You may want to journal regularly. You can confine your journaling to only one topic, such as working through problems in a difficult relationship. You can journal about many things, from the mundane to the extraordinary. You can buy a spiral-bound notebook or a beautifully ornate padded version. You may wish to journal using a password-protected document on your home computer. With the invention of word processing programs, it is quite easy to keep multiple journals, each for a different reason or use.

A journal may be a collection of thoughts, inspirational quotes, relationship "to-do" lists, insights, goals, dreams, and plans. It may be a day-to-day record of what is happening in your inner and outer life. You may record your baby's milestones there, and your ongoing and evolving thoughts on motherhood, womanhood, and selfhood.

Music and Art

As your underlying thoughts and emotions bubble to the surface, you may find it helpful to collect music or art that expresses what you are experiencing. These are also approaches that have been found to be effective in combatting depression (Blomdahl, Gunnarsson, Guregard, & Bjorklund, 2013; Erkkilä, 2011). There is something very affirming about finding that other people can relate to what you are going through, and music and art connect you with the author, the composer, and the artist. Find styles you relate to. Find formats that you will use often and easily, such as a scrapbook, trifold board, MP3 player, or special folder saved on your computer desktop.

If you enjoy drawing, singing, playing an instrument, sewing, quilting, doing crafts, or participating in any other sort of artistic endeavor—indulge yourself in it. Write a story or start a blog. Compose a poem, a song, or a new melody on the guitar. Sketch a picture of your baby, or snap pictures of her using all sorts of background colors and lights. Finish that baby quilt or wall hanging that you put down when the depression took over.

Does it sound like too much? Similar to starting to exercise, just commit yourself to readying your materials and preparing your workspace. Have it all there, waiting for you. Give it five minutes. Until your baby begins to be mobile, which will take several months after her birth, you should be able to leave your materials out between work sessions. If you have older children, you may have to keep your music, art, or sewing materials in a container that is easy for you to access.

It is almost certain that you will be interrupted in any creative activity you begin. This is the reality of motherhood. Just as in your mindfulness practice, where you are learning to tack skillfully between paying attention to internal stimuli and external stimuli, when you are engaged in a project, you learn to tack between attending to your project and attending to the interruptions. The more you master mindfulness, which is the training of the attention, the less frustrating the constant interruptions of motherhood will become. You will be able to be present in your creation of music, art, literature, textiles, or whatever you choose to do. You will also be able to be present in the things that interrupt you.

Psychotherapy

At its essence, psychotherapy is a time and space set aside just for you, for you to work on the issues that you find important. Family and friends have a personal investment in your life, which makes it harder for them to separate your needs from their own. A psychotherapist, by contrast, is a professional trained to help you sort through emotional issues. A psychotherapist also has no personal stake in the decisions you make. This can be very helpful, especially when your longstanding relationship patterns with family members or friends are what you would like to change.

There are various types of psychotherapy and various types of credentials for psychotherapists. In most cases, a psychologist will hold a PhD or PsyD, and be licensed in the jurisdiction where they practice. In some jurisdictions, masters-level therapists can also use the title "psychologist." There are also various other types of therapists: licensed marriage and family therapists (LMFTs), licensed professional counselors (LPCs), and licensed clinical social workers (LCSWs), to name a few. Any of these types of therapists may work for you, if you are able to forge a strong connection with them, and if they are knowledgeable and experienced in treating postpartum depression. It is desirable to find a psychotherapist that specializes in, or at least has experience with, working with depressed new moms. You might check with Postpartum Support International (www. postpartum.net) to see if there are any therapists in your community.

The best way to find out if a therapist is a good fit for you is to meet them or at least to chat with them on the phone. Explain briefly what you are experiencing and ask if this sounds like something they deal with frequently. Some therapists may offer the options of individual or group therapy.

Certain types of psychotherapy have more evidence than others backing up their claims for effectiveness. Cognitive-behavioral therapy, or CBT, and especially CBT that includes a mindfulness component, is one type of psychotherapy with a strong research backing (e.g., Kuyken et al., 2010). Interpersonal therapy (IPT) also has a strong evidence base behind it (Lipsitz & Markowitz, 2013). Ask your potential therapist about the type of treatment that he or she provides and about the evidence base behind it.

Support Groups

You may be able to find support groups through your local hospital or birthing center, or through organizations such as Mothers of Preschoolers International (MOPS), La Leche League (LLL), or Postpartum Support International (PSI). Support groups are different from group therapy, in that they are not usually led by a trained professional and may be more informal. Some situations where a support group may be your best option are when payment for therapy is a concern, when you don't know many other new mothers in your community, when you may not be able to guarantee your attendance at a weekly therapy session, or when your main concern is to become less isolated from others. You may have the opportunity to become a group leader and to pass along what you have learned to others as time goes on. This can be a great feeling and can contribute to your own recovery.

Faith Community

If you are a person of faith, or are considering beginning a faith practice, a faith community, such as a church or synagogue, can provide a ready-made source of personal support. Especially if there are other women who have made it through postpartum depression, and if there is a variety of people ready to love and accept you and your baby, a faith community can be a helping hand on your healing journey. Attendance at worship can be an anchor in a sea of diapers, nighttime feedings, and an otherwise topsy-turvy schedule.

Conclusions

There were many components to my personal recovery from depression. However, I believe that my recovery began the day that

I said this out loud: *I am not going to roll over and let this have me.* I got very, very clear within myself that I have been given only one life, and that it was, and is, up to me to determine what to do with it. I began to create an anchor within myself, an anchor built out of my own experience and my own perspective.

I had to learn to set limits with people. I had to change what I said yes and no to. I had to figure out what I wanted out of life, and how to get it. I had to learn to perceive and accept the things that are my responsibility, and to let go of the things that are not. In some pretty fundamental ways, I had to recreate myself. This took time, partly because I had to learn the principles and skills discussed in this book from scratch and on my own. It also took time simply because that is the nature of lasting change.

You may have read through this chapter and found a reason why you cannot try anything that has been suggested. *I'm too tired. My baby is too fussy. I have no help at home. I have to go back to work too soon.* Living your life just as you always have really is the easiest route. If you are depressed, it is also the more painful route, but it is the easiest. At some point, everyone suffering from depression has to answer the question: *Am I going to roll over and let this have me?*

I hope you fight. I hope you are willing to travel the difficult road that leads to healing. I will be pulling for you.

REFERENCES

Abaied, J., & Emond, C. (2013). Parent psychological control and responses to interpersonal stress in emerging adulthood: Moderating effects of behavioral inhibition and behavioral activation. *Emerging Adulthood, 1*(4), 258-270.

American Psychiatric Association. (2013). *Diagnostic and statistical manual of mental disorders* (5th Ed.). Arlington, VA: American Psychiatric Publishing.

Appolonio, K., & Fingerhut, R. (2008). Postpartum depression in a military sample. *Military Medicine, 173*(11), 1085-1091.

Apted, M. (Director) & Schwartz, B. (Producer). (1980). *Coal Miner's Daughter* [Movie]. Universal City, CA: Universal Pictures.

Asen, E., & Fonagy, P. (2012). Mentalization-based therapeutic interventions for families. *Journal of Family Therapy, 34,* 347-370.

Aube, J. (2008). Balancing concern for other with concern for self: Links between unmitigated communion, communion, and psychological well-being. *Journal of Personality, 76*(1), 101-134.

Barber, B., Xia, M., Olsen, J., McNeely, C., & Bose, K. (2012). Feeling disrespected by parents: Refining the measurement and understanding of psychological control. *Journal of Adolescence, 35,* 273-287.

Baumeister, R., Masicampo, E., & Vohs, K. (2011). Do conscious thoughts cause behavior? *Annual Review of Psychology, 62,* 331-361.

Belsky, J. (2011). Family experience and pubertal development in evolutionary perspective. *Journal of Adolescent Health, 48*(5), 425-426.

Bina, R. (2008). The impact of cultural factors upon postpartum depression: A literature review. *Health Care for Women International, 29*(6), 568-592.

Bokhurst, C., Bakersman-Kranenburg, M., Fearon, R., van Ijzendoorn, M., Fonagy, P., & Schvengel, C. (2003). The importance of shared environment in mother-infant attachment security: A behavioral genetic study. *Child Development, 74*(6), 1769-1782.

Bracha, S., Ralston, T., Matsukawa, J., Williams, A., & Bracha, A. (2004). Does "fight or flight" need updating? *Psychosomatics, 45*(5), 448-449.

Brett, X., Barfield, W., & Williams, C. (2008). Prevalence of self-reported postpartum depressive symptoms: 17 states, 2004-2005. *Morbidity and Mortality Weekly Report, 57*(14), 361-366.

Carlson, D. (2011). Explaining the curvilinear relationship between age at first birth and depression among women. *Social Science and Medicine, 72*, 494-503.

Cassidy, J., & Jones, J. (2014). Parental attachment style: Examination of links with parent secure base provision and adolescent secure base use. *Attachment & Human Development, 16*(5), 437-461.

Centers for Disease Control and Prevention. (2008). Prevalence of self-reported postpartum depressive symptoms—17 states, 2004-2005. *Morbidity and Mortality Weekly Report, 57*(14), 361-366.

Chen, B., & Li, D. (2009). Avoidant strategy in insecure females. *Behavioral and Brain Sciences, 32*(1), 25-26.

Collura, T., Zalaquett, C., Bonnstetter, R., & Chatters, S. (2014). Toward an operational model of decision making, emotional regulation, and mental health impact. *Advances in Mind-Body Medicine, 28*(4), 18-33.

Conway, M. (2005). Memory and the self. *Journal of Memory and Language, 53*(4), 594-628.

Costa, R., & Figueiredo, B. (2011). Infants' psychophysiological profile and temperament at 3 and 12 months. *Infant Behavior and Development, 34*(2), 270-279.

Cuijpers, P., Sijbrandij, M., Koole, S., Andersson, G., Beekman, A., & Reynolds, C. (2014). Adding psychotherapy to antidepressant medication in depression and anxiety disorders: Meta-analysis. *World Psychiatry, 13*, 56-67.

Cutting, A., & Dunn, J. (2002). The cost of understanding other people: Social cognition predicts young children's sensitivity to criticism. *Journal of Child Psychology and Psychiatry, 43*(7), 849-860.

David, D., & Lyons-Ruth, K. (2005). Differential attachment responses of male and female infants to frightening maternal behavior: Tend or befriend versus fight or flight? *Infant Mental Health Journal, 26*(1), 1-18.

De Houwer, J., Barnes-Holmes, D., & Moors, A. (2013). What is learning? On the nature and merits of a functional definition of learning. *Psychonomic Bulletin & Review, 20*(4), 631-642.

Del Giudice, M. (2008), Sex-biased ratio of avoidant/ambivalent attachment in middle childhood. *British Journal of Developmental Psychology, 26*, 369–379.

Del Guidice, M., & Belsky, J. (2010). Sex differences in attachment emerge in middle childhood: An evolutionary hypothesis. *Child Development Perspectives, 4*(2), 97-105.

Dennis, C., & Vigod, S. (2013). The relationship between postpartum depression, domestic violence, childhood violence, and substance use: Epidemiologic study of a large community sample. *Violence Against Women, 19*(4), 503-517.

Desrosiers, A., Vine, V., Klemanski, D., & Nolen-Hoeksema, S. (2013). Mindfulness and emotion regulation in depression and anxiety: Common and distinct mechanisms of action. *Depression and Anxiety, 30*, 654-661.

DiMaggio, G., Salvatore, G., Azzara, C., Catania, D. (2003). Dialogical relationships in impoverished narratives: From theory to clinical practice. *Family Psychology and Psychotherapy, 76*, 385-409.

Dobson, K., Quigley, L., & Dozois, D. (2014). Toward an integration of interpersonal risk models of depression and cognitive-behaviour therapy. *Australian Psychologist, 49*(6), 328-336.

Eberhard-Gran, M., Tambs, K., Opjordsmoen, S., Skrondal, A., & Eskild, A. (2004). Depression during pregnancy and after delivery: A repeated measurement study. *Journal of Psychosomatic Obstetrics and Gynecology, 25*(1), 15-21.

Edwards, M. (2002). Attachment, mastery, and interdependence: A model of parenting processes. *Family Process, 41*(3), 389-404.

Enns, M., Cox, B., & Clara, I. (2002). Parental bonding and adult psychopathology: Results from the U.S. National Comorbidity Survey. *Psychological Medicine, 32*(6), 997-100.

Epkins, C., & Heckler, D. (2011). Integrating etiological models of social anxiety and depression in youth: Evidence for a cumulative risk model. *Clinical Child and Family Psychology Review, 14,* 329-376.

Evraire, L., & Dozois, D. (2011). Qn integrative model of excessive reassurance seeking and negative feedback-seeking in the development and maintenance of depression. *Clinical Psychology Review, 31,* 1291-1303.

Evraire, L., Ludmer, J., & Dozois, A. (2014). The influence of priming attachment styles on excessive reassurance seeking and negative feedback seeking in depression. *Journal of Social and Clinical Psychology, 33*(4), 295-318.

Feldon, D. (2007). Cognitive load and classroom teaching: The double-edged sword of automaticity. *Educational Psychologist, 42*(3), 123-137.

Field, T. (2011). Prenatal depression effects on early development: A review. *Infant Behavior and Development, 34*(1), 1-14.

Fivush, R. (2006). Scripting attachment: Generalized event representations and internal working models. *Attachment & Human Development, 8*(3), 283-289.

Flett, G., Besser, A., Hewitt, P., & Davis, R. (2007). Perfectionism, silencing the self, and depression. *Personality and Individual Differences, 43*(5), 1211-1222.

Galinha, I., Oishi, S., Pereira, C., Wirtz, D., & Esteves, F. (2014). Adult attachment, love styles, relationship experiences, and subjective well-being: Cross-cultural and gender comparisons between Americans, Portuguese, and Mozambicans. *Social Indicators Research, 119*(2), 823-852.

Gausia, K., Fisher, C., Ali, M., & Oosthuizer, J. (2009). Magnitude and contributory factors of postnatal depression: A community-based cohort study from a rural subdistrict of Bangladesh. *Psychological Medicine, 39*(6), 999-1007.

Gill, D., & Warburton, W. (2012). An investigation of the biosocial model of borderline personality disorder. *Journal of Clinical Psychology, 70*(9), 866-873.

Gilbert, P. (2006). Evolution and depression: Issues and implications. *Psychological Medicine, 36,* 287-297.

Gilbert, P., & Gilbert, J. (2003). Entrapment and arrested fight and flight in depression: an exploration using focus groups. *Psychology & Psychotherapy, 76,* 172-188.

Goodman, S., Rouse, M., Connell, A., Broth, M., Hall, C., & Heyward, D. (2011). Maternal depression and child psychopathology: Neonatal depression, a meta-analytic review. *Clinical Child and Family Psychology Review, 14,* 1-27.

Grieve, R. (2011). Mirror mirror: The role of self-monitoring and sincerity in emotional manipulation. *Personality and Individual Differences, 51*(8), 981-985.

Hammen, C. (2005). Stress and depression. *Annual Review of Psychology, 1,* 293-319.

Hammen, C., Shih, J., & Brennan, P. (2004). Intergenerational transmission of depression: Test of an interpersonal stress model in a community sample. *Journal of Consulting and Clinical Psychology, 72*(3), 511-522.

Hankin, B. (2010). Personality and depressive symptoms: Stress generation and cognitive vulnerabilities to depression in a prospective daily diary study. *Journal of Social and Clinical Psychology, 29*(4), 369-401.

Hensch, T. (2004). Critical period regulation. *Annual Review of Neuroscience, 27,* 548-579.

Hill, A., Hall, H., & Appleton, P. (2011). The relationship between multidimensional perfectionism and contingencies of self-worth. *Personality and Individual Differences, 50,* 238-242.

Hogarth, R., & Villeval, M. (2010). *Intermittent reinforcement and the persistence of behavior: Experimental evidence.* Lyon-St. Etienne, France: Groupe d'analyse et de theorie economique.

Immerman, R., & Mackey, W. (2003). The depression gender gap: A view through a biocultural filter. *Genetic, Social, & General Psychology Monographs, 129*(1), 5-39.

Iwaniec, D., Larkin, E., & McSherry, D. (2007). Emotionally harmful parenting. *Child Care in Practice, 13*(3), 203-220.

Jacobvitz, D., Hazen, N., Curran, M., & Hitchens, K. (2004). Observations of early triadic family interactions: Boundary disturbances in the family predict symptoms of depression, anxiety, and attention-deficit/hyperactivity disorder in middle childhood. *Development and Psychopathology, 16*(3), 577-592.

Jin, L., Van Yperen, N., Sanderman, R., & Hagedoorn, M. (2010). Depressive symptoms and unmitigated communion in support providers. *European Journal of Personality, 24,* 56–70.

Jinyao, Y., Xiaongzhao, Z., Auerbach, R., Gardiner, C., Lin, C., Yuping, W., & Shuqiao, Y. (2012). Insecure attachment as a predictor of depressive and anxious symptomatology. *Depression and Anxiety, 29*(9), 789-796.

Johnson, S., Dweck, C., & Chen, F. (2007). Evidence for infants' internal working models of attachment. *Psychological Science, 18*(6), 501-502.

Johnson, D., & Johnson, L. (2010). Reinventing the stress concept. *Ethical Human Psychology and Psychiatry, 12*(3), 218-231.

Jones, T., & Jefferson, S. (2011). Reflections of experience-expectant development in repair of the adult damaged brain. *Developmental Psychobiology, 53,* 468-475.

Joormann, J., & D'Avanzato, C. (2010). Emotion regulation in depression: Examining the role of cognitive processes. *Cognition and Emotion, 24*(6), 913-939.

Julian, C., Wilson, M., & Moore, L. (2009). Evolutionary adaptation to high altitude: A view from in utero. *American Journal of Human Biology, 21*(5), 612-622.

Kang, Y., Gruber, J., & Gray, J. (2013). Mindfulness and de-automatization. *Emotion Review, 5*(2), 192-201.

Kanter, J., Busch, A., Weeks, C., & Landes, S. (2008). The nature of clinical depression: Symptoms, syndromes, and behavior analysis. *The Behavior Analyst/MABA, 31*(1), 1-21.

Kelly, G. (1963). *A theory of personality: The psychology of personal constructs.* New York: W. W. Norton & Company.

Kendall-Tackett, K. (2007). A new paradigm for depression in new mothers: The central role of inflammation and how breastfeeding and anti-inflammatory treatments protect maternal mental health. *International Breastfeeding Journal, 2*(1), 6-6.

Kendall-Tackett, K.A. (2010). *Depression in new mothers, 2nd Ed.* London: Routledge.

Kendall-Tackett, K. (2010). Four research findings that will change the way we think about perinatal depression. *The Journal of Perinatal Education, 19*(4), 7-9.

Kendall-Tackett, K., Cong, Z., & Hale, T. (2011). The effect of feeding method on sleep duration, maternal well-being, and postpartum depression. *Clinical Lactation, 2*(2), 22-26.

Kendler, K., Gardner, C., & Prescott, C. (2006). Toward a comprehensive developmental model for major depression in men. *The American Journal of Psychiatry, 163*(1), 115-124.

Kiff, C., Lengua, L., & Bush, N. (2011). Temperament variation insensitivity to parenting: Predicting changes in depression and anxiety. *Journal of Abnormal Child Psychology, 39*(8), 1199-1212.

Kramer, L., Helmes, A., Seelig, H., Fuchs, R., & Bengei, J. (2014). Correlates of reduced exercise behavior in depression: The role of motivational and volitional deficits. *Psychology and Health, 29*(10), 1206-1225.

Kuyken, W., Watkins, E., Holden, E., White, K., Taylor, R., Byford, S., Evans, A., Radford, S., Teasdale, J., & Dalgleish, T. (2010). How does mindfulness-based cognitive therapy work? *Behaviour Research and Therapy, 48*(11), 1105-1112.

Lawson, C. (2000). *Understanding the borderline mother: Helping her children transcend the intense, unpredictable, and volatile relationship.* Lanham, Maryland: Rowman and Littlefield.

Leach, L., Christensen, H., MacKinnon, A., Windsor, T., & Butterworth, P. (2008). Gender differences in depression and anxiety across the adult lifespan: The role of psychosocial mediators. *Social Psychiatry and Epidemiology, 43,* 983-998.

Lebreton, M., Jorge, S., Michel, V., Thirione, B., & Pessiglioni, M. (2009). An automatic valuation system in the human brain: Evidence from functional neuroimaging. *Neuron, 64*(3), 431-439.

Lecompte, V., & Moss, E. (2014). Disorganized and controlling patterns of attachment, role reversal, and caregiving helplessness: Links to adolescents' externalizing problems. *American Journal of Orthopsychiatry, 84*(5), 581-589.

Lefkovics, E., Baji, I., & Rigo, J. (2014). Impact of maternal depression on pregnancies and on early attachment. *Infant Mental Health Journal, 35*(4), 354-365.

Lehnart, J., Penke, L., Asendorpf, J., & Neberich, W. (2010). Family of origin, age at menarche, and reproductive strategies: A test of four evolutionary-developmental models. *European Journal of Developmental Psychology, 7*(2), 153-177.

Levitt, H., Frankel, Z., Hiestano, K., Ware, K., Bretz, K., Kelly, R., McGhee, S., Nordtvedt, R., & Raina, K. (2004). The transformational experience of insight: A life-changing event. *Journal of Constructivist Psychology, 17*(1), 1-26.

Lipsitz, J., & Markowitz, J. (2013). Mechanisms of change in interpersonal therapy (IPT). *Clinical Psychology Review, 33*(8), 1134-1147.

McCullough, J., James, P., Lord, B., Martin, A., Conley, K., Schramm, E., & Klein, D. N. (2011). The significant other history: An interpersonal-emotional history procedure used with the early-onset chronically depressed patient. *American Journal of Psychotherapy, 65*(3), 225.

McDonald, K., Bowker, J., Rubin, K., Laursen, B., & Duchene, M. (2010). Interactions between rejection sensitivity and supportive relationships in the prediction of adolescents' internalizing difficulties. *Journal of Youth and Adolescence, 39,* 563-574.

McKenna, J., & McDade, T. (2005). Why babies should never sleep alone: A review of the co-sleeping controversy in relation to SIDS, bedsharing, and breast feeding. *Paediatric Respiratory Reviews, 6,* 134-152.

McKenzie, L., Purvis, K., & Cross, D. (2014). A trust-based intervention for special needs adopted children: A case study. *Journal of Aggression, Maltreatment, and Trauma, 23*(6), 633-651.

McWilliams, S. (2013). A 21st-century personal construct psychology upgrade. *Journal of Constructivist Psychology, 26*(3), 164-171.

Meites, T., Ingram, R., & Siegle, G. (2012). Unique and shared aspects of affective symptomatology: The role of parental bonding in depression and anxiety symptom profiles. *Cognitive Therapy and Research, 36,* 173-181.

Messman-Moore, T., & Coates, A. (2007). The impact of childhood psychological abuse on adult interpersonal conflict. *Journal of Emotional Abuse, 7*(2), 75-92.

Mills, R., Freeman, W., & Clara, I. (2007). Parent proneness to shame and the use of psychological control. *Journal of Child and Family Studies, 16*(3), 359.

Morris, M., Evans, L., Rao, U., & Garber, J. (2015). Executive function moderates the relation between coping and depressive symptoms. *Anxiety, Stress, and Coping, 28*(1), 31-49.

Nagurney, A. (2008). The effects of unmitigated communion and life events among women with fibromyalgia syndrome. *Journal of Health Psychology, 13,* 520-528.

Newman, C. (2010). The case of Gabriel: Treatment with Beckian cognitive therapy. *Journal of Constructivist Psychology, 23*(1), 25-41.

O'Mahen H.A., Flynn H.A., & Nolen-Hoeksema S.N. (2010). Rumination and interpersonal functioning in perinatal depression. *Journal of Social and Clinical Psychology, 29*(6), 646-667.

Nylen, K., Moran, T., Franklin, C., & O'Hara, M. (2006). Maternal depression: A review of relevant approaches for mothers and infants. *Infant Mental Health Journal, 27*(4), 327-343.

Otani, K., Suzuki, A., Matsumoto, Y., Shibuya, N., Sadaniro, R., & Enokido, M. (2013). Parental overprotection engenders dysfunctional attitudes about achievement and dependency in a gender-specific manner. *BMC Psychiatry, 13,* 345-349.

Ottenbreit, N. D., Dobson, K.S., & Quigley, L. (2014). An examination of avoidance in major depression in comparison to social anxiety disorder. *Behaviour Research and Therapy, 56,* 82-90.

Overbeek, G., ten Have, M., Vollebergh, W., & de Graaf, R. (2007). Parental lack of care and overprotection: Longitudinal associations with DSM-III-R disorders. *Social Psychiatry and Psychiatric Epidemiology, 42*(2), 87-93.

Perry, J. C., Sigal, J. J., Boucher, S., & Paré, N. (2006). Seven institutionalized children and their adaptation in late adulthood: The children of duplessis *(les enfants de duplessis). Psychiatry, 69*(4), 283-301.

Raison, C., Jain, R., Maletic, V., & Draud, J. (2009). From chaos to consilience: Part III: What the new mind-body science tells us about the pathophysiology of major depression—focus on treatment. *Psychiatric Times, 26*(8), 25-27.

Raison, C., & Miller, A. (2013). The evolutionary significance of depression in Pathogen Host Defense (PATHOS-D). *Molecular Psychiatry, 18,* 15-37.

Raskin, J. (2013). Thinking, feeling, and being human. *Journal of Constructivist Psychology, 26*(3), 181-186.

Ribeiro, A., Sousa, I., Angus, L., Mendes, I., Gonçalves, M., & Stiles, W. (2014). Ambivalence in emotion-focused therapy for depression: The maintenance of problematically dominant self-narratives. *Psychotherapy Research, 24*(6), 702-710.

Riva, G., Gaudio, S., & Dakanalis, A. (2014). The neuropsychology of self-objectification. *European Psychologist, 1*(1), 1-10.

Roelofs, K., Hagenaars, M., & Stins, J. (2004). Facing freeze: Social threat induces body freeze in humans. *Psychological Science, 21*(11), 1575-1581.

Sakaluk, J. (2014). Problems with recall-based attachment style priming paradigms: Exclusion criteria, sample bias, and reduced power. *Journal of Social and Personal Relationships, 31*(7), 888-906.

Saunders, R., Jacobovitz, D., Zaccagnino, M., Beuerung, L., & Hazen, N. (2011). Pathways to earned security: The role of alternative support figures. *Attachment and Human Development, 13*(4), 403-420.

Scheber, T. (2011). Evolutionary psychology, cognitive function, and deterrence. *Comparative Strategy, 30*(5), 453-480.

Sedikides, C., & Green, J. (2004). What I don't recall can't hurt me: Information negativity versus information inconsistency as determinants of memorial self-defense. *Social Cognition, 22*(1), 4-29.

Seligman, M., & Maier, S. (1967). Failure to escape traumatic shock. *Journal of Experimental Psychology, 74*(1), 1-9.

Shenk, C., & Fruzzetti, A. (2014). Parental validating and invalidating responses and adolescent psychological functioning: An observational study. *The Family Journal: Counseling and Therapy for Couples and Families, 22*(1), 43-48.

Silverstein, M., & Ruiz, S. (2006). Breaking the chain: How grandparents moderate the transmission of maternal depression to their grandchildren. *Family Relations, 55*(5), 601-612.

Sorenson, D., & Tschetter, L. (2010). Prevalence of negative birth perception, disaffirmation, perinatal trauma symptoms, and depression among postpartum women. *Perspectives in Psychiatric Care, 46*(1), 14-25.

Sroufe, A. (2013). The promise of developmental psychopathology: Past and present. *Development and Psychopathology, supplement: Development and Psychopathology: A Vision Realized, 25*(4, part 2), 1215-1224.

Steel, P. (2007). The nature of procrastination: A meta-analytic and theoretical review of quintessential self-regulatory failure. *Psychological Bulletin, 133*(1), 65-94.

Szymanski, D., Moffitt, L., & Carr, E. (2011). Sexual objectification of women: Advances to theory and research. *The Counseling Psychologist, 39*(1), 6-38.

Tambling, R. (2012). A literature review of therapeutic expectancy effects. *Contemporary Family Therapy, 34*(3), 402-415.

Tan, J., & Carfagnini, B. (2008). Self-silencing, anger and depressive symptoms in women: Implications for prevention and intervention. *Journal of Prevention and Intervention in the Community, 35*(2), 5-18.

Taylor, S. (2006). Tend and befriend: Biobehavioral bases of affiliation under stress. *Current Directions in Psychological Science, 15*(6), 273-277.

Thompson, K., & Bendell, D. (2014). Depressive cognitions, maternal attitudes and postnatal depression. *Journal of Reproductive and Infant Psychology, 32*(1), 70-82.

Toomey, B., & Ecker, B. (2007). Of neurons and knowledge: Constructivism, coherence, psychology, and their neurodynamic substrates. *Journal of Constructivist Psychology, 20*(3), 201-245.

Ussher, J. (2004). Premenstrual syndrome and self-policing: Ruptures in self-silencing leading to increased self-surveillance and blaming of the body. *Social Theory and Health, 2*(3), 254-271.

Vliegen, N., & Luyten, P. (2008). The role of dependency and self-criticism in the relationship between postpartum depression and anger. *Personality and Individual Differences, 45,* 34-40.

Veale, D. (2008). Behavioural activation for depression. *Advances in Psychiatric Treatment, 14*(1), 29-36.

Wei, C., & Kendall, P. (2004). Parental involvement: Contribution to childhood anxiety and its treatment. *Clinical Child and Family Psychology Review, 17,* 319-339.

Wigley, S. (2007). Automaticity, consciousness, and moral responsibility. *Philosophical Psychology, 20*(2), 209-225.

Wise, T., Fishbain, D., & Holder-Perkins, V. (2007). Painful physical symptoms in depression: A clinical challenge. *Pain Medicine, 8*(2), 75-82.

Worlein, J. (2014). Nonhuman primate models of depression: Effects of early experience and stress. *ILAR Journal, 55*(2), 259-273.

Yap, M., Allen, N., & Ladouceur, C. (2008). Maternal socialization of positive affect: The impact of invalidation on adolescent emotion regulation and depressive symptomatology. *Child Development, 79*(5), 1415-1431.

Yirmiya, R., Pollak, Y., Morag, M., Reichenberg, A., Barak, O., Avitsur, R., Shavit, Y., Ovadia, H., Weidenfeld, J., Morag, A., Newman, M., & Pollmacher, T. (2000). Illness, cytokines, and depression. *Annals of the New York Academy of Sciences, 917*(1), 478-487.

Zelkowitz, P., Saucier, J., Wang, T., Katofsky, L., Valenzuela, M., & Westreich, R. (2008). Stability and change in depressive symptoms from pregnancy to two months postpartum in childbearing immigrant women. *Archives of Women's Mental Health, 11,* 1-11.

Zuroff, D., Fournier, M., & Moskowitz, D. (2007). Depression, perceived inferiority, and interpersonal behavior: Evidence for the involuntary defeat strategy. *Journal of Social and Clinical Psychology, 26*(7), 751-778.

Made in the USA
Middletown, DE
04 June 2016